Transforming Healthcare with Big Data

Healthcare organizations are utilizing big data for improved data analytics and performance measurements. This book provides a comprehensive framework integrating 41 components, emphasizing data completeness for better healthcare outcomes. It provides guidelines for selecting appropriate technology and implementing solutions.

Transforming Healthcare with Big Data: A Practical Guide for Big Data in Healthcare Systems presents a six-layer framework for healthcare systems, integrating organization, people, process, data, technology, and outcomes. It discusses big data analytics, predictive risk assessments, and the benefits of combining it with artificial intelligence, machine learning, and deep learning technologies. It also guides planning big data analytics solutions, tracking KPIs, and optimizing healthcare operations for cost reduction without compromising care quality.

Healthcare executives, administrators, IT professionals, data scientists, analysts, clinical and operations managers, consultants, researchers, academics, policymakers, and graduate students in health informatics and industrial engineering can all benefit from this book by gaining a comprehensive and practical framework for effectively implementing big data analytics in healthcare. This will enable improved patient outcomes, cost efficiency, and operational excellence.

Transforming Healthcare with Big Data

A Practical Guide for Big Data in Healthcare Systems

Ahmed Mohamed, Luis Rabelo,
and Juan Pablo Zamora-Aguas

CRC Press
Taylor & Francis Group
Boca Raton London New York

CRC Press is an imprint of the
Taylor & Francis Group, an Informa business

First edition published 2026
by CRC Press
2385 NW Executive Center Drive, Suite 320, Boca Raton FL 33431

and by CRC Press
4 Park Square, Milton Park, Abingdon, Oxon, OX14 4RN

CRC Press is an imprint of Taylor & Francis Group, LLC

Library of Congress Cataloging-in-Publication Data
Names: Mohamed, Ahmed, PhD author | Rabelo Mendizabal, Luis C. (Luis Carlos), 1960- author | Zamora-Aguas, Juan Pablo author
Title: Transforming healthcare with big data : a practical guide for big data in healthcare systems / Ahmed Mohamed, Luis Rabelo and Juan Pablo Zamora-Aguas.
Description: First edition. | Boca Raton FL : CRC Press, 2026. | Includes bibliographical references.
Identifiers: LCCN 2025030272 (print) | LCCN 2025030273 (ebook) | ISBN 9781041005391 hardback | ISBN 9781041006046 paperback | ISBN 9781003610731 ebook
Subjects: LCSH: Medical informatics | Big data
Classification: LCC R859.7.D35 M64 2026 (print) | LCC R859.7.D35 (ebook)
LC record available at https://lccn.loc.gov/2025030272
LC ebook record available at https://lccn.loc.gov/2025030273

ISBN: 978-1-041-00539-1 (hbk)
ISBN: 978-1-041-00604-6 (pbk)
ISBN: 978-1-003-61073-1 (ebk)

DOI: 10.1201/9781003610731

Typeset in Times
by KnowledgeWorks Global Ltd.

Dedication

Mohamed Ahmed wants to dedicate this book to Mohamed family.

Luis Rabelo wants to dedicate this book to his sons, Luis Gisli and Carlos Magnus.

Juan Pablo Zamora wants to dedicate this book to his wife, Giovanna, and his son, Juan Esteban.

Contents

Preface

TRANSFORMING HEALTHCARE WITH BIG DATA: A PRACTICAL GUIDE FOR BIG DATA IN HEALTHCARE SYSTEMS

Healthcare organizations (HCOs) currently have many information about their patients. Yet, they often cannot make proper, faster, and more thoughtful conclusions with their information. Much of the information, such as historical and non-clinical medical records, is structured. This data is stored in a central repository called the data warehouse (DW). DW provides querying and reporting to different groups within the HCO to support their future strategic initiatives.

Additionally, HCOs seek to benefit from semi-structured and unstructured data by adopting emerging technology such as big data to aggregate all collected data from different sources obtained from electronic medical records (EMR), scheduling, registration, billing systems, and wearable devices into one volume for better data analysis. For data completeness, big data is essential to improving healthcare systems. It is expected to revamp the outlook of the healthcare industry by reducing costs and improving quality.

This book presents a framework for utilizing big data that interconnects all aspects of healthcare for real-time analytics and performance measurements. It is a comprehensive framework that integrates 41 integrated components in six layers—Organization, People, Process, Data, Technology, and Outcomes—to ensure successful implementation. Each component in the framework and its linkage with other components are explained to show coherence. Moreover, it highlights how data completeness leads to better healthcare quality outcomes, and it is essential for HCOs' survival.

In this book, the framework offers guidelines for selecting the appropriate technology with the flexibility of implementing the solution on a small or large scale, considering the benefits vs. investment. It revealed that focusing only on big data technology could cause a failed implementation without accomplishing the desired value of the data analytics outcomes. It is only applied to one-dimensional, not at the enterprise level.

The book is intended for leaders of HCOs to understand the future of healthcare utilizing big data and analytics toward the fourth revolution in healthcare, known as Healthcare 4.0 (H 4.0). The content of the book covers the following fundamental subjects:

- **Big Data and Healthcare Information Technology (HIT)**
- **Healthcare Systems and Data Mapping**
- **Big Data Analytics Framework**
- **Case Study—Implementation of Big Data Analytics**
- **The future of healthcare with emerging technology**

The value creation of big data analytics in healthcare came because of the forced demands in the industry to make a positive impact using innovation with data and new emerging technology. Big data feeds other analytics technologies, such as deep learning, machine learning, and Artificial Intelligence (AI), that can help HCOs achieve better outcomes. Thus, big data won't be useful without AI and ML, and vice versa. AI, DL, and ML cannot fully take advantage of data completeness, including big data.

Introduction

The convergence of data science and healthcare represents one of the most transformative shifts in modern medicine. As the global healthcare industry grapples with rising costs, fragmented systems, and increasing demands for personalized care, the emergence of big data offers both a formidable challenge and an unprecedented opportunity. *Transforming Healthcare with Big Data* arrives at a critical juncture—bridging the gap between theoretical potential and practical implementation.

What distinguishes this book is its thoughtful integration of systems thinking, healthcare operations, and cutting-edge data technologies. Built around a comprehensive six-layer framework—Organization, People, Processes, Data, Technology, and Outcomes—the book offers a structured path for healthcare institutions to transition from legacy systems to real-time, insight-driven ecosystems. It draws on principles from Healthcare 4.0, systems engineering, and industrial analytics to create a blueprint that is scalable, adaptable, and evidence based.

The book presents real-world case studies, validated frameworks, and lessons from experienced subject matter experts (SMEs), all culminating in a practical guide for executives, IT professionals, data scientists, and policy leaders. From the fragmented origins of clinical and operational data to the deployment of generative AI, the authors chart a course through the complex terrain of digital transformation in healthcare.

This is not merely a book about technology, it is a guide to organizational renewal. By addressing governance, workforce readiness, data quality, and strategic alignment, it speaks to the human and systemic dimensions of innovation. It is a call to action for healthcare leaders to embrace analytics not just as a tool, but as a culture—new way of thinking, working, and healing.

With this book, we offer a contribution to the global healthcare community—one grounded in vision, practical insight, and a commitment to advancing care through data. Whether you are initiating your digital transformation journey or refining established infrastructures, we hope this guide serves as a lasting resource—both as a roadmap for action and as a catalyst for innovation. Our intent is to empower professionals across the healthcare spectrum to realize the full potential of big data, transforming systems into more intelligent, resilient, and patient-centered.

The Authors!

About the Authors

Ahmed Mohamed, PhD, is currently the Director of Solutions Engineering at Orlando Health, Orlando, Florida, with 25-plus years of technical and management experience in Information Technology and Healthcare. Additionally, he has been involved in teaching graduate courses at Webster University at the Orlando Campus as an Adjunct Instructor. He received his PhD and MS degrees in Industrial Engineering from the Department of Industrial Engineering and Management Systems (IEMS), University of Central Florida, Orlando, Florida. He also earned an MS degree from City College of New York in 1994 and his BS degree from Alexandria University, Alexandria, Egypt, in 1990, all in Electrical Engineering. Dr. Mohamed holds several certifications, including PMP, CLSSBB, CSM, ITIL V3, and a Graduate Certificate for Quality Assurance. His focus is on healthcare process improvements by utilizing information technology and data analytics.

Luis Rabelo, PhD, was the NASA EPSCoR Agency Project Manager and is currently a Professor in the Department of IEMS at the University of Central Florida, Orlando, Florida. He received a joint degree in Electrical and Mechanical Engineering from Panama and a master's degree from the Florida Institute of Technology, Melbourne, Florida (1987) and the University of Missouri, Columbia, Missouri (1988). He received a PhD in Engineering Management from the University of Missouri, Columbia, Missouri, in 1990, where he also did post-doctoral work in Nuclear Engineering (1991). In addition, Dr. Rabelo holds a dual MS degree in Systems Engineering & Management from the Massachusetts Institute of Technology, Cambridge, Massachusetts, and has over 300 publications, 3 international patents, and has graduated 60 doctoral students as advisors/co-advisors to his credit.

Juan Pablo Zamora-Aguas, MSc, is currently pursuing his doctoral studies in Industrial Engineering at the University of Central Florida, Orlando, Florida. He earned his degree in Industrial Engineering (2002) and a postgraduate degree in Engineering Project Management (2005) from the Francisco José de Caldas District University, Bogotá, Colombia. He received his Master's degree in Industrial Engineering with honors from the National University of

Colombia, Bogotá, Colombia (2014). Juan Pablo has been active in academia since 2006, holding various roles as a Lecturer, Part-Time Professor, and Full-Time Professor. For the past 10 years, he served as a Full-Time Professor at the University of La Salle, Bogotá, Colombia. He has led research projects and participated in consulting teams for government institutions in Colombia, focusing on pharmaceutical supply chain management, quality management in pharmacy service, and other areas of healthcare management using risk analysis and system dynamics.

Acknowledgments

We would like to express our deepest appreciation to the many individuals and organizations whose contributions were instrumental in developing this book.

We are also grateful to the **University of Central Florida**, particularly the **Department of Industrial Engineering and Management Systems**, for providing an environment that encourages interdisciplinary research and the integration of engineering principles with healthcare applications. The department's ongoing dedication to data-driven systems helped shape the foundation of this book.

Finally, we sincerely thank Taylor & Francis for publishing this book and for their infinite patience. We are confident that this work represents a valuable contribution to the evolving landscape of healthcare transformation and the strategic use of big data to drive intelligent, patient-centered systems.

The Promise and Challenge of Big Data in Healthcare

1

1.1 A NEW ERA OF HEALTHCARE INTELLIGENCE

Healthcare is undergoing a profound transformation, driven by the rapid expansion of data in volume, variety, velocity, and veracity. Providers, including hospitals, clinics, labs, pharmacies, insurance, and practitioners, generate vast amounts of patient information daily from sources such as electronic medical records (EMRs), electronic health records (EHRs), billing systems, diagnostic imaging, lab tests, patient-reported outcomes, and wearable devices. This growing digital ecosystem now includes behavioral health data, social determinants of health (SDoH), and consumer-generated inputs like fitness trackers and mobile health apps.

Yet much of this data remains trapped in fragmented systems and diverse structured, semi-structured, and unstructured formats, hindering timely analysis and insight. This fragmentation limits healthcare organizations' ability to make informed decisions that could enhance care, efficiency, and population health.

Big data is central to this shift: datasets are too large, complex, or fast moving for traditional tools. Defined by the "5 Vs"—volume, velocity, variety, veracity, and value—big data in healthcare spans sensor outputs, genomic data, clinical notes, and insurance claims. Its true promise lies not just in scale but in uncovering patterns, generating predictions, and enabling intelligent automation.

DOI: 10.1201/9781003610731-1

When combined with artificial intelligence (AI), including machine learning (ML) and natural language processing (NLP), big data powers a shift from retrospective reporting to real-time, predictive intelligence. This enables impactful applications like clinical decision support, risk stratification, proactive care coordination, early detection, revenue optimization, and personalized medicine.

This book presents a strategic framework to harness big data's full potential in healthcare. Built around six core pillars—organization, people, processes, data, technology, and outcomes—it supports the transition to insight-driven, adaptive enterprises aligned with the principles of healthcare 4.0. By embedding analytics into operations, aligning data with strategy, and creating interoperable platforms, healthcare systems can deliver faster, smarter, and more equitable care, prepared for today's challenges and tomorrow's opportunities.

1.2 A CRISIS OF COMPLEXITY AND COST

Despite significant technological advancements, the US healthcare system grapples with structural challenges. As of 2025, the United States continues to lead globally in healthcare spending, reaching $4.9 trillion in 2023, representing 17.6% of the nation's gross domestic product (GDP)—projected to rise to nearly 20% by 2032 (McGough et al., 2024). Despite this substantial investment, the United States continues to underperform in key health outcomes. In 2023, life expectancy at birth was 78.4 years, approximately 4.1 years lower than the average among other high-income countries (McGough et al., 2024). Moreover, despite having the highest per capita health expenditures, the US healthcare system ranks last among 11 high-income nations regarding access, equity, and health outcomes (Etienne, 2024). This misalignment between spending and outcomes underscores the urgent need for systemic reforms to enhance efficiency, equity, and overall population health.

One of the most pressing issues is the underutilization of vast healthcare data, particularly semi-structured data such as physician notes and unstructured formats including scanned images, PDFs, and free-text narratives. These valuable data sources often remain siloed and disconnected from enterprise-wide decision-making tools.

The fragmentation of performance measurement systems compounds the problem. Financial, operational, and clinical departments often operate in isolation, each maintaining separate key performance indicators (KPIs) that do not align into a unified, actionable framework. The lack of a centralized, real-time analytics infrastructure significantly hinders healthcare providers' ability to make informed decisions quickly, optimize operations, and enhance patient outcomes.

1.3 THE PROBLEM WE MUST SOLVE

At the heart of the challenge lies a dependence on manual processes and the inaccessibility of critical data. Semi-structured and unstructured data, such as physician notes, scanned documents, and free-text records, are often reviewed manually by healthcare personnel. This consumes valuable time and introduces variability and a higher risk of human error. Despite the vast data, healthcare organizations frequently lack the tools and infrastructure to generate timely, actionable insights that inform clinical and operational decisions.

This reality prompts a pressing question: *How can we develop a robust framework that leverages big data technologies and advanced analytics to unlock real-time value from complex, fragmented healthcare data, transforming it into a strategic asset rather than an underused burden?*

1.4 OBJECTIVES AND VISION

This book aims to introduce a scalable and flexible framework that will:

- unify disparate data sources (structured, semi-structured, and unstructured),
- enable real-time analytics that inform clinical and operational decisions,
- develop KPIs grounded in data completeness,
- reduce costs and improve quality of care through intelligent performance monitoring, and
- empower organizations to comply with evolving government regulations

1.5 A CONTRIBUTION TO HEALTHCARE 4.0

While many existing big data models in healthcare focus on narrow clinical applications or specific technologies, they often overlook broader organizational and systemic needs. This book presents a holistic framework grounded in Healthcare 4.0 principles—leveraging cyber-physical systems, Internet of Things (IoT), AI, and advanced analytics to build an intelligent, connected, patient-centered ecosystem.

Rooted in systems engineering and Industrial Engineering principles, the framework prioritizes interoperability, scalability, and enterprise alignment. It integrates technologies like cloud computing, data lakes, and AI-driven analytics while embedding governance, workflows, and workforce readiness to ensure sustainable transformation.

Modular and adaptable, the framework can be applied incrementally or on a scale, making it suitable for diverse healthcare settings—from small clinics to integrated health systems. Ultimately, it serves as both a strategic blueprint and a practical guide, enabling healthcare organizations to evolve from reactive operations to intelligent, data-driven platforms that support personalized care, proactive risk management, and continuous performance improvement.

1.6 SCOPE AND LIMITATIONS

The healthcare industry is inherently complex. Unlike conventional industries, where costs, services, and transactions are typically transparent and standardized, healthcare processes frequently involve ambiguity in pricing, reimbursement, and service delivery responsibilities. This lack of clarity presents significant challenges to developing and implementing universally standardized frameworks.

The proposed framework in this book is designed to serve as a comprehensive foundation for leveraging big data analytics in healthcare performance measurement. However, it is not intended as a rigid, one-size-fits-all solution. Rather, it should be regarded as a modular and adaptable blueprint tailored to meet various healthcare environments' specific needs, maturity levels, and operational realities. The framework provides a strategic starting point for driving data-informed transformation, whether applied in large hospital systems, outpatient facilities, academic research centers, or integrated delivery networks.

1.7 WHAT LIES AHEAD

The remainder of this book guides readers through the conceptual, analytical, and practical journey that shaped the proposed big data analytics framework for healthcare:

- **Chapter 2** reviews the literature and theoretical foundations, identifying key gaps between current capabilities and desired outcomes in healthcare performance measurement.
- **Chapter 3** titled Leveraging Big Data and Analytics for Predictive Risk Assessment and KPIs outlines the research methodology, including insights from literature review, case studies, data analysis, and expert interviews across various healthcare settings.
- **Chapter 4** details the proposed framework, explaining its six pillars—organization, People, Processes, Data, Technology, and Outcomes—and how 41 interconnected components drive scalable, insight-driven transformation.
- **Chapter 5** presents real-world validation, comparing manual and automated analytics to assess efficiency, accuracy, and decision-making gains.
- **Chapter 6** synthesizes key insights and discusses the broader impact of big data and AI in healthcare. It highlights Healthcare 4.0 trends such as generative AI while underscoring the importance of transparency, fairness, privacy, and accountability.

REFERENCES

Etienne, V. (2024). United States healthcare system ranks last among fellow wealthy countries, new report says: "Dramatically lower." In *People*. https://people.com/united-states-healthcare-system-ranks-last-report-8715530

McGough, M., Winger, A., Kurani, N., & Cox, C. (2024). How much is health spending expected to grow? In *Peterson-KFF Health System Tracker*. https://www.healthsystemtracker.org/chart-collection/how-much-is-health-spending-expected-to-grow/

Insights and Gaps in Big Data Analytics in Healthcare

2

2.1 INTRODUCTION

The deepening concern for offering patient-centered healthcare added to the increasing development of big data analytics technologies has intensified the interest to implement comprehensive systems to manage valuable data in healthcare environments. Healthcare organizations generate vast amounts of data that include patient medical records in electronic format, patient tracking and patient monitoring, records of text communication of discharge summaries, and imaging. As well as medical data, relevant operations data on the healthcare management is generated permanently. Making sense of data and using it appropriately has led to the implementation of several applications opening important paths in the provision of medical services supported by technology. Factors associated with patient healthcare have been used to perform predictive modelling of disease trends, disease detection, and personalized treatment which has demonstrated substantial benefits for patient health. This is very closely related to the possibility of focusing health efforts and resources based on data and its analysis through technology.

From a point of view of healthcare management, the adoption of technological developments in big data analytics pursues favorable outcomes on overall performance of healthcare organizations. For example, simulation with real-time data on operational and human resources enables impactful decision-making process. The integration of core and supportive

DOI: 10.1201/9781003610731-2

processes in healthcare through big data analytics strategy generates capabilities that strengthen the healthcare services and improve the organizational performance.

Big data analytics (BDA) is a multidisciplinary field interconnected with a broad spectrum of knowledge and technologies (Ü. Demirbaga et al., 2024). BDA is supported by a wide range of platforms and tools. IT infrastructure, distributed computing, statistics, and applied mathematics have a strong connection with artificial intelligence (AI) and machine learning.

In Section 2.1, the methodology of the literature review and the bibliographic analysis are presented. Section 2.2 is focused on the state of art where trends in the main fields on big data analytics in healthcare are presented. In Section 2.3 a comprehensive analysis of insights is discussed. In Section 2.4 conclusions and connection with the other chapters are presented.

2.2 LITERATURE REVIEW METHODOLOGY

The methodology adopted to perform the literature review was founded on the PRISMA 2020 statement (Page et al., 2021). The literature search strategy was developed using two broad terms aligned with the objective of the review, enabling an analysis of the results in relation to the key questions. The combination of words for the bibliographic search strategy corresponded to: "big data analytics" and "healthcare". Web of Science, IEEE Xplore, and Pubmed databases were used for the searches. All terms were applied to the field Topic in the Web of Science database; Title/Abstract in the Pubmed, and Abstract in the IEEE Xplore. All results were combined into a single record, and duplicates were removed. The process of identification, selection, and inclusion of articles is presented in Table 2.1. In total 1378 records were found. Review articles, editorial material, letters, retracted publications, meeting abstracts were not included. Articles in languages other than English, articles with insufficient information, and articles that do not correspond to the research topic were discarded. The period of publications found in this search ranges from 2000 to 2024. However, due to the low number of articles published until 2012, the analysis period was taken between 2013 and 2024. The number of articles used for the bibliographic analysis was 812.

TABLE 2.1 PRISMA 2020-based study identification and inclusion summary

PHASE	*DESCRIPTION*	*NUMBER OF RECORDS*
Identification	**Records Identified from**:	
	Web of Science	891
	IEEE Xplore	301
	PubMed	231
	Records Removed before Screening:	
	• Duplicates removed	327
	• Records marked as ineligible	201
Screening	Records screened	895
	Records excluded	83
Eligibility	**Records Used for Bibliographic Analysis Using Bibliometrix**	812
	Reports excluded:	
	• Thematic connection	193
	• PageRank measure	561
Included	**Studies Included in Review**	58
	Qualitative synthesis	18

2.2.1 Bibliometric Analysis

Bibliometric analysis enables the discovery of insights, the identification of trends, and the detection of knowledge gaps in the literature. The conceptual structure was analyzed through thematic evolution and thematic map visualizations using Bibliometrix R package (Aria & Cuccurullo, 2017). Both visualizations allow the grouping of the main themes through clusters. While clusters are created based on the dynamic trajectory of research themes for the thematic evolution, showing how they emerge, persist, or decline over time, thematic map clusters are generated through a cohesive group of keywords at a single point in time without showing changes over time (Cobo et al., 2011).

2.2.1.1 Thematic evolution

For the thematic evolution analysis, three time slices were defined. As seen in Table 2.2, the first time slice corresponds to articles published between 2013

TABLE 2.2 Thematic evolution for bigrams of abstracts

2013–2017	*2018–2021*	*2022–2024*
Performance measurements	Data analytics	Data analytics
Healthcare providers	Cloud computing	Supply chain
Data analytics	Patient outcomes	Machine learning
Decision support	Supply chain	Health organizations
Cloud computing	Machine learning	Social media
Patient data	Structural equation	
Claims data	Performance measurement	
Proposed architecture	Data technology	
Data applications	Smart grid	

and 2017, the second for the period between 2018 and 2021, and the third covers publications between 2022 and 2024. This table presents the dominant research themes, identified through the co-occurrence analysis of terms extracted as bigrams from abstracts across the defined time periods.

These topics reflect a growing research interest in technology integration and data-driven strategies that are transforming the delivery and management of healthcare services. A more detailed analysis reveals relationships of direct continuity when themes persist over time, such as data analytics or supply chain management. Thematic fusion occurs when several themes evolve and converge, contributing to the development of new research topics, models, or applications. For example, technological advancements in cloud computing have facilitated the use of web applications and social media. Thematic transformation occurs when a topic evolves, generating new paradigms or areas of research interest, such as machine learning and artificial intelligence.

2.2.1.2 Thematic map

A thematic map was used to analyze the conceptual structure of the research domain within the entire period of the bibliographic base found. Thematic maps group related keywords, terms, or topics in the literature into clusters based on their co-occurrence in the analyzed articles. This visualization provides a representation of themes/clusters based on their relevance degree giving by centrality, and their development degree giving by density (Aria et al., 2020). The thematic maps classify themes/clusters in four categories (Cobo et al., 2011). First, motor themes correspond to important and well-developed

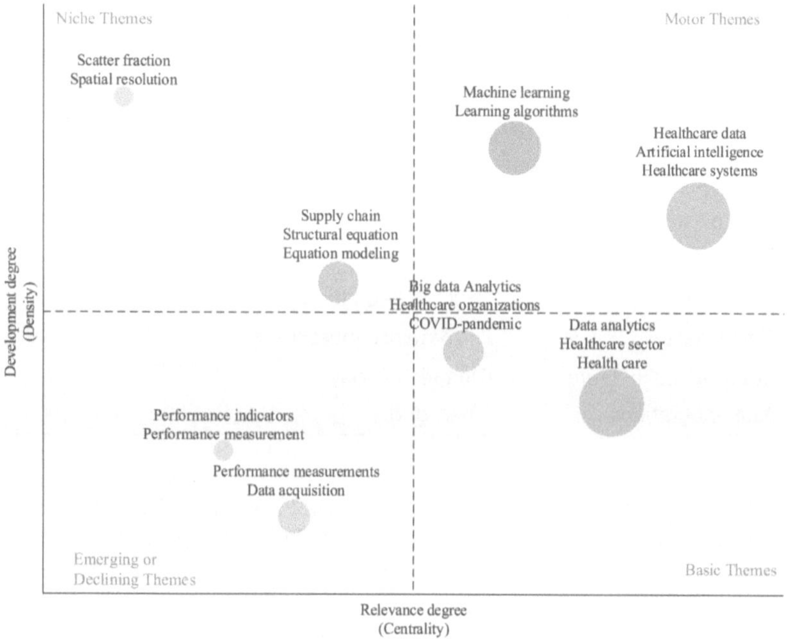

FIGURE 2.1 Thematic map using Bibliometrix for bigrams of abstracts 2013–2024.

themes that have high centrality and high density. Then, the niche themes are specialized but not broadly connected themes. Their main characteristics are low centrality and high density. Thirdl, emerging or declining themes are weakly developed themes, potentially growing or fading. These present low centrality and low density. Finally, basic themes represent general or fundamental topics with broad connections but limited development. Their main characteristics are high centrality and low density. Eight clusters were generated in the thematic map, as shown in Figure 2.1.

2.3 STRUCTURAL ANALYSIS OF LITERATURE THEMES AND CONTEXTS

Based on the bibliographic analysis, Figure 2.2 illustrates the thematic structure of the reviewed literature, including key topics, thematic clusters, subclusters, and their respective classifications. The illustration is

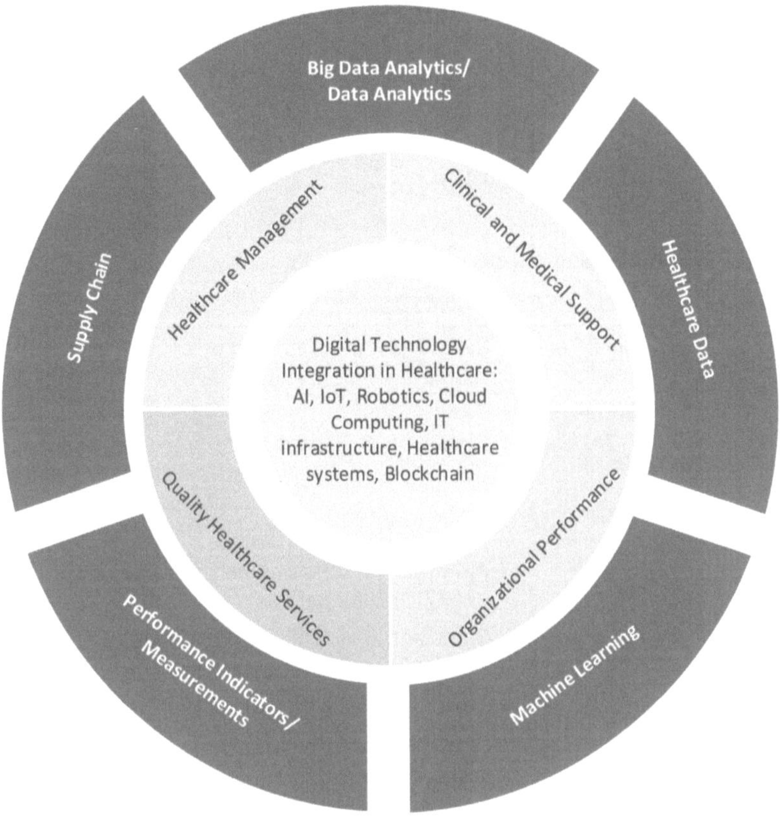

FIGURE 2.2 Thematic structure of big data analytics in healthcare.

designed as follows. The outer rings correspond to the main topics or clusters derived from the bibliographic analysis. The term with the highest frequency of occurrence was assigned to the cluster name based on the centrality and density analysis of the thematic map analysis. The central ring corresponds to subclusters or subtopics in the general scope of the research.

These subtopics were defined based on the application context observed in the literature and correspond to healthcare management, clinical and medical support, organizational performance, and quality healthcare services. The core of the graph presents the main technologies reported in the literature. Their relationship with the application context (central ring) is observed from their contributions of the literature.

2.3.1 Main Contributions in the Literature

Below, for each cluster and subcluster, the subjects addressed by the most representative authors in each topic are presented. The criterion used to select the authors corresponded to the PageRank measure. The topics addressed in each cluster are shown in Tables 2.3–2.7.

TABLE 2.3 Main contributions in the big data/data analytics cluster

CLUSTER	*SUBCLUSTER*	*ARTICLE*	*SUBJECTS*
Big data/Data analytics	Clinical and medical domains	Neves and Burgers (2022)	Telemedicine; primary care; quality of care
		Yang et al. (2022)	Smart E-health services; smart healthcare management system (SHMS); multi-criteria decision-making (MCDM)
		Wu et al. (2017)	Bioinformatics; -Omic data; precision medicine
		Gupta and Kumar (2023)	Artificial intelligence; precision medicine; neurological disorders
		Geldof et al. (2019)	Oncology; data exploring; federated network
		Vallée (2024)	Otorhinolaryngology; digital twin; artificial intelligence; personalized medicine
		Jan et al. (2024)	Wearable devices; artificial intelligence of medical things; (AIOMT); internet of medical things (IOMT)
Big data/Data analytics	Healthcare management	Wang et al. (2018)	Big data analytics capabilities; business value of information technology (IT)
		Wang and Hajli (2017)	Capability building view; resource-based theory
		Edu (2024)	IOTs; configural paths; FSQCA
		Korayim et al. (2024)	Competitive advantage; organizational innovation; data driven culture

(*Continued*)

TABLE 2.3 Main contributions in the big data/data analytics cluster (*Continued*)

CLUSTER	*SUBCLUSTER*	*ARTICLE*	*SUBJECTS*
		Akter et al. (2024)	Analytics empowerment capability; humanitarian analytics
		Shahbaz et al. (2019)	Big data analytics; healthcare; trust
		Batko and Ślęzak (2022)	Data-driven healthcare; big data; big data analytics
		El Samad et al. (2022)	Data quality; data cleaning; data correction; decision-making
Big data/Data analytics	Organizational performance	Sousa et al. (2019)	Decision-making; leaders; business intelligence
		Wang et al. (2018)	IT-Enabled transformation; practice-based view; business value of IT
		Yu et al. (2023)	Hospitals; medical services; decision-making; big data analytics capability (BDAC)
		Saha and Rathore (2024)	Healthcare 4.0 technologies; hospital supply chain processes
Big data/ Data analytics	Quality healthcare services	Basile et al. (2024)	Digital transformation; risk management; decision-making

TABLE 2.4 Main contributions in the healthcare data cluster

CLUSTER	*SUBCLUSTER*	*ARTICLE*	*SUBJECTS*
Healthcare data	Clinical and medical functions	Ali et al. (2021)	Healthcare monitoring system; wearable sensors; social network analysis
		Safa et al. (2023)	Diabetes; blood pressure, sensor, IoT devices; decisive support systems
		Manogaran et al. (2018)	Wearable medical devices; wireless sensor networks; internet of things; cloud computing
		Srinivas et al. (2020)	Biomedical monitoring; medical services; wearable sensors

(*Continued*)

TABLE 2.4 Main contributions in the healthcare data cluster (*Continued*)

CLUSTER	*SUBCLUSTER*	*ARTICLE*	*SUBJECTS*
Healthcare data	Healthcare management	Li et al. (2021)	Sensing; big data; data analytics; internet of things
		Demirbaga and Aujla (2022)	Medical services; blockchain; cloud computing; internet of things
		Ristevski and Chen (2018)	Data mining; health informatics; healthcare information systems
Healthcare data	Quality healthcare services	Batarseh and Latif (2016)	Quality of service; big data analytics; healthcare; forecasting
		Zhang et al. (2017)	Patient-centric applications and services; body area networks (Bans); big data; cloud computing; cyber-physical systems (CPS)

TABLE 2.5 Main contributions in the machine learning cluster

CLUSTER	*SUBCLUSTER*	*ARTICLE*	*SUBJECTS*
Machine learning	Clinical and medical functions	Fancy et al. (2025)	Disease diagnosis; Hadoop Mapreduce; big data
		Asri and Jarir (2023)	Miscarriage prediction; predictive analytics; clustering
		Kumar and Sunitha (2024)	Disease diagnosis; map reduce; chaotic red deer optimizer; deep learning; hyperparameter tuning
		Awotunde et al. (2024)	Breast cancer; bioinformatics; deep convolutional neural network; ant colony optimization
		Khatibi et al. (2022)	Apgar score prediction; distributed feature selection; distributed classification; stack ensemble
		Lambay and Mohideen (2024)	Cardio disease prediction; feature selection; supervised machine learning; drug recommendation

(*Continued*)

TABLE 2.5 Main contributions in the machine learning cluster (*Continued*)

CLUSTER	*SUBCLUSTER*	*ARTICLE*	*SUBJECTS*
		Chen et al. (2017)	Prediction of chronic disease outbreak, big data analytics; machine learning
		Hadi et al. (2020)	Stroke out-patients (OPS) Hetnet uplink optimization; MILP; patient-centric; network optimization; resource allocation
		Geo Jenefer and Deepa (2023)	Diabetes disease prediction; Catboost (Cb); feature scaling
		Kanchanamala et al. (2023)	Heart disease prediction; Shepard convolutional neural network; horse herd optimization
		Hu et al. (2018)	Aided diagnosis for outpatient; spatio-temporal evolution
		Moreira et al. (2018)	Gestational diabetes; computational intelligence; decision-making; artificial neural networks

TABLE 2.6 Main contributions in the performance measurements/performance indicators cluster.

CLUSTER	*SUBCLUSTER*	*ARTICLE*	*SUBJECTS*
Performance measurements/ Performance indicators	Organizational performance	Peng et al. (2007)	Intellectual capital; performance measurement (quality); health services; Taiwan
		Scorza et al. (2022)	Benchmarking; crowding solution; emergency department (ED) crowding; length of stay (LOS); performance EDs measure
Performance measurements/ Performance indicators	Quality healthcare services	Cho et al. (2020)	Process performance indicators; process mining; emergency room; healthcare; performance measurements
		Saez et al. (2018)	Intelligent healthcare management; artificial intelligence; big data

TABLE 2.7 Main contributions in the supply chain cluster

CLUSTER	*SUBCLUSTER*	*ARTICLE*	*SUBJECTS*
Supply chain	Organizational performance	Wantao Yu et al. (2021)	Hospital supply chain integration; operational flexibility; organizational information processing theory
		Surajit Bag et al. (2023)	Omnichannel; healthcare business; artificial intelligence; big data analytics
		Bag et al. (2024)	Medical services; responsive supply chain; supply chain innovation; supply chain resilience
		Benzidia et al. (2021)	Big data analytics; AI; environmental performance; green supply chain process
		Furstenau et al. (2022)	Healthcare digitalization; smart supply chain; resilience; healthcare supply chain
		Benzidia et al. (2024)	Big data analytics capability; green innovation; operations; environmental performance
		Tiwari et al. (2024)	Supply chain visibility; environmental dynamism; healthcare supply chain resilience
		Chatterjee et al. (2023)	Artificial intelligence; Industry 4.0; healthcare supply chain performance; supply chain resilience; sustainability
Supply chain	Quality healthcare services	Desingh and Baskaran (2022)	Quality of patient care; fuzzy MICMAC; Indian healthcare; internet of things; interpretive structural modeling (ISM)
		Smith et al. (2024)	Safety; quality; healthcare supply chain
		Srivastava and Singh (2021)	ISCP; patient centricity; healthcare; service delivery; antecedents; relationships
		van de Wetering (2021)	Patient service performance; digital dynamic capability; patient agility; hospitals

2.4 RESEARCH GAP ANALYSIS

The bibliographic analysis revealed several significant research gaps in the intersection of data management, analytics, and healthcare systems. These gaps highlight critical areas where current literature is either underdeveloped or lacks practical integration, particularly in the context of complex, data-driven health environments.

2.4.1 Context-Specific Data Models in Healthcare

While numerous studies discuss data models and frameworks, few are explicitly tailored to specific healthcare contexts such as primary care, hospital management, or public health surveillance. This lack of contextualization limits the practical applicability of generic models, which often fail to address the unique data flows, regulatory requirements, and stakeholder needs present in distinct healthcare environments. Developing data models that align with the operational realities of these settings is essential to support effective decision-making and enhance service delivery.

2.4.2 Performance Measurement and KPIs from a Systemic Perspective

Existing performance measurement approaches in healthcare often focus narrowly on clinical outcomes or financial indicators. There is a notable gap in comprehensive, systemic performance frameworks that integrate key performance indicators (KPIs) across multiple levels, including service quality (e.g., patient satisfaction, accessibility), organizational health management (e.g., leadership effectiveness, process integration), strategic level (e.g., alignment with health policy goals), operational level (e.g., resource utilization, logistics, workflow optimization), and technological level (e.g., IT system reliability, data interoperability). Addressing this gap is critical for enabling holistic performance evaluations that support continuous improvement and alignment with healthcare objectives.

2.4.3 Big Data Models for Healthcare Applications

Although big data is a growing topic in healthcare research, there remains a deficiency in robust models that can effectively harness large-scale, heterogeneous datasets (e.g., EHRs, imaging data, wearable sensors, social determinants of health). The absence of standardized, scalable big data frameworks impedes the ability to generate actionable insights, predict trends, and personalize care at scale.

2.4.4 Data Warehousing Architectures

The literature reveals limited exploration of how traditional and modern data warehousing architectures such as data warehouses, marts, and lakes are being applied or adapted in healthcare settings. These architectures are crucial for data integration, historical analysis, and supporting business intelligence tools. A better understanding and documentation of their implementation in healthcare can support scalable, flexible, and cost-effective data ecosystems.

2.4.5 Cloud-Based Data Hosting Solutions

Despite the increasing adoption of cloud computing in other sectors, its strategic use in healthcare data hosting remains insufficiently studied. Research is lacking on cloud-based architectures that ensure compliance with data privacy regulations (e.g., Health Insurance Portability and Accountability Act (HIPAA), General Data Protection Regulation (GDPR)), support real-time analytics, and facilitate interoperability across systems and institutions. Exploring this area is vital for enabling agile, secure, and collaborative health information systems.

These gaps represent critical barriers to the effective use of data and analytics in healthcare decision-making. Addressing them can lead to improved design and implementation of data-driven healthcare strategies, enhanced operational efficiency and resource management, better patient outcomes through tailored performance metrics and predictive modeling, and more scalable and interoperable health information infrastructures. By filling these gaps, future research can contribute to building smarter, more resilient, and value-based healthcare systems.

REFERENCES

Akter, S., Motamarri, S., Sajib, S., Bandara, R. J., Tarba, S., & Vrontis, D. (2024). Theorising the microfoundations of analytics empowerment capability for humanitarian service systems. *Annals of Operations Research*, *335*(3), 989–1013. https://doi.org/10.1007/s10479-021-04386-5

Ali, F., El-Sappagh, S., Islam, S. M. R., Ali, A., Attique, M., Imran, M., & Kwak, K.-S. (2021). An intelligent healthcare monitoring framework using wearable sensors and social networking data. *Future Generation Computer Systems*, *114*, 23–43. https://doi.org/10.1016/j.future.2020.07.047

Aria, M., & Cuccurullo, C. (2017). Bibliometrix: An R-tool for comprehensive science mapping analysis. *Journal of Informetrics*, *11*(4), 959–975. https://doi.org/10.1016/j.joi.2017.08.007

Aria, M., Misuraca, M., & Spano, M. (2020). Mapping the evolution of social research and data science on 30 years of social indicators research. *Social Indicators Research*, *149*(3), 803–831. https://doi.org/10.1007/s11205-020-02281-3

Asri, H., & Jarir, Z. (2023). Toward a smart health: Big data analytics and IoT for real-time miscarriage prediction. *Journal of Big Data*, *10*(1), 34. https://doi.org/10.1186/s40537-023-00704-9

Awotunde, J. B., Panigrahi, R., Shukla, S., Panda, B., & Bhoi, A. K. (2024). Big data analytics enabled deep convolutional neural network for the diagnosis of cancer. *Knowledge and Information Systems*, *66*(2), 905–931. https://doi.org/10.1007/s10115-023-01971-x

Bag, S., Dhamija, P., Singh, R. K., Rahman, M. S., & Sreedharan, V. R. (2023). Big data analytics and artificial intelligence technologies based collaborative platform empowering absorptive capacity in health care supply chain: An empirical study. *Journal of Business Research*, *154*, 113315. https://doi.org/10.1016/j.jbusres.2022.113315

Bag, S., Gupta, S., Choi, T.-M., & Kumar, A. (2024). Roles of innovation leadership on using big data analytics to establish resilient healthcare supply chains to combat the COVID-19 pandemic: A multimethodological study. *IEEE Transactions on Engineering Management*, *71*, 13213–13226. https://doi.org/10.1109/TEM.2021.3101590

Basile, L. J., Carbonara, N., Panniello, U., & Pellegrino, R. (2024). The role of big data analytics in improving the quality of healthcare services in the Italian context: The mediating role of risk management. *Technovation*, *133*, 103010. https://doi.org/10.1016/j.technovation.2024.103010

Batarseh, F. A., & Latif, E. A. (2016). Assessing the quality of service using big data analytics: With application to healthcare. *Big Data Research*, *4*, 13–24. https://doi.org/10.1016/j.bdr.2015.10.001

Batko, K., & Ślęzak, A. (2022). The use of big data analytics in healthcare. *Journal of Big Data*, *9*(1), 3. https://doi.org/10.1186/s40537-021-00553-4

Benzidia, S., Bentahar, O., Husson, J., & Makaoui, N. (2024). Big data analytics capability in healthcare operations and supply chain management: The role of green process innovation. *Annals of Operations Research*, *333*(2), 1077–1101. https://doi.org/10.1007/s10479-022-05157-6

Benzidia, S., Makaoui, N., & Bentahar, O. (2021). The impact of big data analytics and artificial intelligence on green supply chain process integration and hospital environmental performance. *Technological Forecasting and Social Change*, *165*, 120557. https://doi.org/10.1016/j.techfore.2020.120557

Chatterjee, S., Chaudhuri, R., Gupta, S., Mangla, S. K., & Kamble, S. (2023). Examining the influence of industry 4.0 in healthcare supply chain performance: Moderating role of environmental dynamism. *Journal of Cleaner Production*, *427*, 139195. https://doi.org/10.1016/j.jclepro.2023.139195

Chen, M., Hao, Y., Hwang, K., Wang, L., & Wang, L. (2017). Disease prediction by machine learning over big data from healthcare communities. *IEEE Access*, *5*, 8869–8879. https://doi.org/10.1109/ACCESS.2017.2694446

Cho, M., Song, M., Park, J., Yeom, S.-R., Wang, I.-J., & Choi, B.-K. (2020). Process mining-supported emergency room process performance indicators. *International Journal of Environmental Research and Public Health*, *17*(17). https://doi.org/10.3390/ijerph17176290

Cobo, M. J., López-Herrera, A. G., Herrera-Viedma, E., & Herrera, F. (2011). An approach for detecting, quantifying, and visualizing the evolution of a research field: A practical application to the fuzzy sets theory field. *Journal of Informetrics*, *5*(1), 146–166. https://doi.org/10.1016/j.joi.2010.10.002

Demirbaga, U., & Aujla, G. S. (2022). MapChain: A blockchain-based verifiable healthcare service management in IoT-based big data ecosystem. *IEEE Transactions on Network and Service Management*, *19*(4), 3896–3907. https://doi.org/10.1109/TNSM.2022.3204851

Demirbaga, Ü, Aujla, G. S., Jindal, A., & Kalyon, O.. (2024). Big Data Analytics Platforms. In Ü. Demirbaga, G. S. Aujla, A. Jindal, & O. Kalyon (Eds.), *Big data analytics: Theory, techniques, platforms, and applications* (pp. 79–126). Springer Nature Switzerland. https://doi.org/10.1007/978-3-031-55639-5_5

Desingh, V., & Baskaran, R. (2022). Internet of things adoption barriers in the Indian healthcare supply chain: An ISM-Fuzzy MICMAC approach. *The International Journal of Health Planning and Management*, *37*(1), 318–351. https://doi.org/10.1002/hpm.3331

Edu, A. S. (2024). Configural paths for IoTs and big data analytics acceptance for healthcare improvement: A fuzzy-set qualitative comparative analysis. *Aslib Journal of Information Management*, *76*(5), 800–821. https://doi.org/10.1108/AJIM-10-2022-0465

El Samad, M., El Nemar, S., Sakka, G., & El-Chaarani, H. (2022). An innovative big data framework for exploring the impact on decision-making in the European Mediterranean healthcare sector. *EuroMed Journal of Business*, *17*(3), 312–332. https://doi.org/10.1108/EMJB-11-2021-0168

Fancy, C., Krishnaraj, N., Ishwarya, K., Raja, G., & Chandrasekaran, S. (2025). Modelling of healthcare data analytics using optimal machine learning model in big data environment. *Expert Systems*, *42*(1), e13612. https://doi.org/10.1111/exsy.13612

Furstenau, L. B., Zani, C., Terra, S. X., Sott, M. K., Choo, K.-K. R., & Saurin, T. A. (2022). Resilience capabilities of healthcare supply chain and supportive digital technologies. *Technology in Society*, *71*, 102095. https://doi.org/10.1016/j.techsoc.2022.102095

Geldof, T., Huys, I., & Van Dyck, W. (2019). Real-world evidence gathering in oncology: The need for a biomedical big data insight-providing federated network. *Frontiers in Medicine, 6*. https://doi.org/10.3389/fmed.2019.00043

Geo Jenefer, G., & Deepa, A. J. (2023). Diabetes disease prediction using firefly optimization-based cat-boost classifier in big data analytics. *Journal of Intelligent & Fuzzy Systems, 44*(6), 9943–9954. https://doi.org/10.3233/JIFS-223105

Gupta, N. S., & Kumar, P. (2023). Perspective of artificial intelligence in healthcare data management: A journey towards precision medicine. *Computers in Biology and Medicine, 162*, 107051. https://doi.org/10.1016/j.compbiomed.2023.107051

Hadi, M. S., Lawey, A. Q., El-Gorashi, T. E. H., & Elmirghani, J. M. H. (2020). Patient-centric HetNets powered by machine learning and big data analytics for 6g networks. *IEEE Access, 8*, 85639–85655. https://doi.org/10.1109/ACCESS.2020.2992555

Hu, Y., Duan, K., Zhang, Y., Hossain, M. S., Mizanur Rahman, S. M., & Alelaiwi, A. (2018). Simultaneously aided diagnosis model for outpatient departments via healthcare big data analytics. *Multimedia Tools and Applications, 77*(3), 3729–3743. https://doi.org/10.1007/s11042-016-3719-1

Jan, M. A., Zhang, W., Akbar, A., Song, H., Khan, R., & Chelloug, S. A. (2024). A hybrid mutual authentication approach for artificial intelligence of medical things. *IEEE Internet of Things Journal, 11*(1), 311–320. https://doi.org/10.1109/JIOT.2023.3317292

Kanchanamala, P., Alphonse, A. S., & Reddy, P. V. B. (2023). Heart disease prediction using hybrid optimization enabled deep learning network with spark architecture. *Biomedical Signal Processing and Control, 84*, 104707. https://doi.org/10.1016/j.bspc.2023.104707

Khatibi, T., Farahani, A., Sepehri, M. M., & Heidarzadeh, M. (2022). Distributed big data analytics method for the early prediction of the neonatal 5-minute apgar score before or during birth and ranking the risk factors from a national dataset. *AI, 3*(2), 371–389. https://doi.org/10.3390/ai3020023

Korayim, D., Chotia, V., Jain, G., Hassan, S., & Paolone, F. (2024). How big data analytics can create competitive advantage in high-stake decision forecasting? The mediating role of organizational innovation. *Technological Forecasting and Social Change, 199*, 123040. https://doi.org/10.1016/j.techfore.2023.123040

Kumar, R. H., & Sunitha, G. (2024). Big data analytics in healthcare environment using chaotic red deer optimizer with deep learning for disease classification model. *Multimedia Tools and Applications, 83*(32), 77697–77715. https://doi.org/10.1007/s11042-024-18239-3

Lambay, M. A., & Mohideen, S. P. (2024). Applying data science approach to predicting diseases and recommending drugs in healthcare using machine learning models – A cardio disease case study. *Multimedia Tools and Applications, 83*(26), 68341–68361. https://doi.org/10.1007/s11042-023-18035-5

Li, W., Chai, Y., Khan, F., Jan, S. R. U., Verma, S., Menon, V. G., Kavita, & Li, X. (2021). A comprehensive survey on machine learning-based big data analytics for IoT-enabled smart healthcare system. *Mobile Networks and Applications, 26*(1), 234–252. https://doi.org/10.1007/s11036-020-01700-6

Manogaran, G., Varatharajan, R., Lopez, D., Kumar, P. M., Sundarasekar, R., & Thota, C. (2018). A new architecture of internet of things and big data ecosystem for secured smart healthcare monitoring and alerting system. *Future Generation Computer Systems, 82*, 375–387. https://doi.org/10.1016/j.future.2017.10.045

Moreira, M. W. L., Rodrigues, J. J. P. C., Kumar, N., Al-Muhtadi, J., & Korotaev, V. (2018). Evolutionary radial basis function network for gestational diabetes data analytics. *Journal of Computational Science, 27*, 410–417. https://doi.org/10.1016/j.jocs.2017.07.015

Neves, A. L., & Burgers, J. (2022). Digital technologies in primary care: Implications for patient care and future research. *European Journal of General Practice, 28*(1). https://doi.org/10.1080/13814788.2022.2052041

Page, M. J., McKenzie, J. E., Bossuyt, P. M., Boutron, I., Hoffmann, T. C., Mulrow, C. D., Shamseer, L., Tetzlaff, J. M., Akl, E. A., Brennan, S. E., Chou, R., Glanville, J., Grimshaw, J. M., Hróbjartsson, A., Lalu, M. M., Li, T., Loder, E. W., Mayo-Wilson, E., McDonald, S., & Moher, D.. (2021). The PRISMA 2020 statement: An updated guideline for reporting systematic reviews. *The BMJ, 372*. https://doi.org/10.1136/bmj.n71

Peng, T. A., Pike, S., & Roos, G. (2007). Intellectual capital and performance indicators: Taiwanese healthcare sector. *Journal of Intellectual Capital, 8*(3), 538–556. https://doi.org/10.1108/14691930710774902

Ristevski, B., & Chen, M. (2018). Big data analytics in medicine and healthcare. *Journal of Integrative Bioinformatics, 15*(3). https://doi.org/10.1515/jib-2017-0030

Saez, Y., Gómez, A. B., Rada, & de, F. (2018). DataCare: Big data analytics solution for intelligent healthcare management. *International Journal of Interactive Multimedia and Artificial Intelligence, 4*(Special Issue on Big Data and e-Health), 13–20. http://www.ijimai.org/journal/sites/default/files/files/2017/03/ijimai_4_7_2_pdf_16566.pdf

Safa, M., Pandian, A., Gururaj, H. L., Ravi, V., & Krichen, M. (2023). Real time health care big data analytics model for improved QoS in cardiac disease prediction with IoT devices. *Health and Technology, 13*(3), 473–483. https://doi.org/10.1007/s12553-023-00747-1

Saha, E., & Rathore, P. (2024). The impact of healthcare 4.0 technologies on healthcare supply chain performance: Extending the organizational information processing theory. *Technological Forecasting and Social Change, 201*, 123256. https://doi.org/10.1016/j.techfore.2024.123256

Scorza, A., Porazzi, E., Strozzi, F., Garagiola, E., Gimigliano, A., & De Filippis, G. (2022). A new approach for emergency department performance positioning: The quality-efficiency matrix. *The International Journal of Health Planning and Management, 37*(3), 1636–1649. https://doi.org/10.1002/hpm.3428

Shahbaz, M., Gao, C., Zhai, L., Shahzad, F., & Hu, Y. (2019). Investigating the adoption of big data analytics in healthcare: the moderating role of resistance to change. *Journal of Big Data, 6*(1), 6. https://doi.org/10.1186/s40537-019-0170-y

Smith, S., Lane, M., Toleman, M., & Shrestha, A. (2024). Safety and quality within the healthcare supply chain: A great unknown. *Studies in Health Technology and Informatics, 310*, 364–368. https://doi.org/10.3233/SHTI230988

Sousa, M. J., Pesqueira, A. M., Lemos, C., Sousa, M., & Rocha, Á (2019). Decision-Making based on big data analytics for people management in healthcare organizations. *Journal of Medical Systems*, *43*(9), 290. https://doi.org/10.1007/s10916-019-1419-x

Srinivas, J., Das, A. K., Kumar, N., & Rodrigues, J. J. P. C. (2020). Cloud centric authentication for wearable healthcare monitoring system. *IEEE Transactions on Dependable and Secure Computing*, *17*(5), 942–956. https://doi.org/10.1109/TDSC.2018.2828306

Srivastava, S., & Singh, R. K. (2021). Exploring integrated supply chain performance in healthcare: A service provider perspective. *Benchmarking: An International Journal*, *28*(1), 106–130. https://doi.org/10.1108/BIJ-03-2020-0125

Tiwari, M., Bryde, D. J., Stavropoulou, F., Dubey, R., Kumari, S., & Foropon, C. (2024). Modelling supply chain visibility, digital technologies, environmental dynamism and healthcare supply chain resilience: An organisation information processing theory perspective. *Transportation Research Part E: Logistics and Transportation Review*, *188*, 103613. https://doi.org/10.1016/j.tre.2024.103613

Vallée, A. (2024). Challenges and directions for digital twin implementation in otorhinolaryngology. *European Archives of Oto-Rhino-Laryngology*, *281*(11), 6155–6159. https://doi.org/10.1007/s00405-024-08662-5

van de Wetering, R. (2021). *Achieving Digital-Driven Patient Agility in the Era of Big Data BT – Responsible AI and Analytics for an Ethical and Inclusive Digitized Society* (D. Dennehy, A. Griva, N. Pouloudi, Y. K. Dwivedi, I. Pappas & M. Mäntymäki (eds.); pp. 82–93). Springer International Publishing. https://doi.org/10.1007/978-3-030-85447-8_8

Wang, Y., & Hajli, N. (2017). Exploring the path to big data analytics success in healthcare. *Journal of Business Research*, *70*, 287–299. https://doi.org/10.1016/j.jbusres.2016.08.002

Wang, Y., Kung, L., Wang, W. Y. C., & Cegielski, C. G. (2018). An integrated big data analytics-enabled transformation model: Application to health care. *Information & Management*, *55*(1), 64–79. https://doi.org/10.1016/j.im.2017.04.001

Wang, Y., Kung, L. A., & Byrd, T. A. (2018). Big data analytics: Understanding its capabilities and potential benefits for healthcare organizations. *Technological Forecasting and Social Change*, *126*, 3–13. https://doi.org/10.1016/j.techfore.2015.12.019

Wu, P.-Y., Cheng, C.-W., Kaddi, C. D., Venugopalan, J., Hoffman, R., & Wang, M. D. (2017). –Omic and electronic health record big data analytics for precision medicine. *IEEE Transactions on Biomedical Engineering*, *64*(2), 263–273. https://doi.org/10.1109/TBME.2016.2573285

Yang, C.-H., Hsu, W., & Wu, Y.-L. (2022). A hybrid multiple-criteria decision portfolio with the resource constraints model of a smart healthcare management system for public medical centers. *Socio-Economic Planning Sciences*, *80*, 101073. https://doi.org/10.1016/j.seps.2021.101073

Yu, W., Liu, Q., Zhao, G., & Song, Y. (2023). Exploring the effects of data-driven hospital operations on operational performance from the resource orchestration theory perspective. *IEEE Transactions on Engineering Management*, *70*(8), 2747–2759. https://doi.org/10.1109/TEM.2021.3098541

Yu, W., Zhao, G., Liu, Q., & Song, Y. (2021). Role of big data analytics capability in developing integrated hospital supply chains and operational flexibility: An organizational information processing theory perspective. *Technological Forecasting and Social Change*, *163*, 120417. https://doi.org/10.1016/j.techfore.2020.120417

Zhang, Y., Qiu, M., Tsai, C.-W., Hassan, M. M., & Alamri, A. (2017). Health-CPS: Healthcare cyber-physical system assisted by cloud and big data. *IEEE Systems Journal*, *11*(1), 88–95. https://doi.org/10.1109/JSYST.2015.2460747

3 Leveraging Big Data and Analytics for Predictive Risk Assessment and KPIs

3.1 KEY ASPECTS FROM RESEARCH METHODOLOGY

3.1.1 Research Idea

Several technologies that are recently introduced to the business community such as machine learning, deep learning, artificial intelligence (AI), and big data are going to change the outlook of the healthcare industry as well as other related fields. The goal is to explore these technologies to lead to breakthrough approaches that are necessary to solve the issues of high cost and enhance the quality outcomes in healthcare. It is expected numerous research focus on the healthcare industry to take advantage of big data features of dealing with images, handwriting, and texts in unstructured data format and to find innovative solutions to help healthcare leaders be proactive with real-time data in their decision-making.

The idea of the research is to architect a solution utilizing big data technology to enhance the performance measurements of the healthcare system.

DOI: 10.1201/9781003610731-3

A survey of literature is conducted to find the proposed ideas to accomplish the goal of improving the performance measurement of the healthcare systems and to present the literature gap that identify the missing key points for better optimizations in both quality and cost of the healthcare system.

3.1.2 Analysis from Survey of Literature

Based on the literature review, it is possible to identify various areas of research interest related to big data analytics and healthcare. According to the bibliometric analysis presented in Chapter 2, five key clusters of interest have emerged in which the literature has contributed to advancing knowledge in this field: big data analytics, healthcare data, machine learning, performance indicators/measurements, and supply chain management.

To develop this chapter, appropriate future research questions have been formulated within the context of performance, which is considered a critical aspect of health systems from a systemic perspective. The importance of the performance component in health management lies in the broad range of areas it encompasses. Specifically, the literature review's thematic structure highlights performance in clinical and medical support areas, organizational performance, health service quality, and healthcare management.

3.1.3 Gap Analysis

The literature reveals several gaps in key areas of healthcare data and performance. These include the need for context-specific data models, as well as improved methods for measuring performance and defining KPIs from a systemic perspective. Each of these areas plays a critical role in shaping the overall performance of healthcare management. A comprehensive view of performance shows that these gaps affect not only the quality of healthcare services but also strategic planning, support operations, and the use of technology. In light of these findings, it is important to propose future research questions and explore possible approaches to address these gaps. Table 3.1 shows nine research questions for future works and the approaches for the big data in healthcare performance measurements.

Hence, the research question "how big data technologies help automating the search of needed performance measurements utilizing semi-structured and unstructured data in real-time and accuracy outcomes in healthcare?" is validated as an identified gap.

TABLE 3.1 Research gap analysis (part 1)

GAP DESCRIPTION	*RESEARCH QUESTIONS FOR FUTURE WORKS*	*POSSIBLE APPROACHES*
Context-specific data models in healthcare (Korayim et al., 2024; Demirbaga & Aujla, 2022; Hadi et al., 2020; Yu et al., 2021)	1. *How can data models be tailored to fit the operational workflows of primary care, hospitals, or public health agencies?* 2. *What are the unique data requirements and regulatory constraints in each healthcare context?* 3. *How do stakeholder roles affect data model design in different settings?*	Conduct case studies in different healthcare environments Co-design with domain experts and end users Develop modular, adaptable data modeling frameworks Use domain-driven design (DDD) methodologies
Performance measurement and KPIs from a systemic perspective (Cho et al., 2020; Scorza et al., 2022; Benzidia et al., 2024; Chatterjee et al., 2023)	4. *What integrated frameworks can capture performance across clinical, operational, strategic, and technological levels?* 5. *How can KPIs be linked across multiple layers of healthcare systems to support systemic evaluation?* 6. *How do systemic KPIs influence decision-making and quality improvement?*	Design multi-level KPI frameworks Apply systems thinking and performance management approaches Use simulation and modeling to test KPI interrelations Pilot integrated dashboards in real-world settings
Big data models for healthcare applications (Fancy et al., 2025; Asri & Jarir, 2023; Kumar & Sunitha, 2024; Awotunde et al., 2024)	7. *What scalable models can effectively integrate and analyze heterogeneous healthcare data sources?* 8. *How can big data models support predictive analytics and personalized care?* 9. *What standards and architectures are needed to ensure data quality and interoperability at scale?*	Develop big data pipelines using frameworks like Apache Spark, Hadoop Employ data fusion and deep learning techniques Create ontology-based integration models Establish standards-based interoperability protocols (e.g., FHIR)

Healthcare as an industry is a very sophisticated business and it has several issues in many aspects including high cost and lack of quality. Adopting digital transformation in healthcare has helped improving the overall experience for both patients and caregivers.

TABLE 3.2 Research gap analysis (part 2)

GAP DESCRIPTION	*RESEARCH QUESTIONS FOR FUTURE WORKS*	*POSSIBLE APPROACHES*
Data warehousing architectures (Wang et al., 2018; Hoque et al., 2024; Ristevski & Chen, 2018)	1. *How are data warehousing solutions currently deployed in healthcare environments?* 2. *What are the advantages and challenges of using warehouses, marts, or lakes for different healthcare data types?* 3. *How can warehousing architectures support historical analysis and real-time BI?*	Comparative analysis of different warehousing approaches in healthcare Design reference architectures for specific healthcare use cases Incorporate hybrid models combining warehouse and lake paradigms Evaluate using real-world data integration case studies
Cloud-based data hosting solutions (Jan et al., 2024; Aqeel et al., 2023; Demirbaga & Aujla, 2022)	4. *How can cloud-based solutions comply with strict healthcare data privacy regulations?* 5. *What architectures support real-time analytics and interoperability in the cloud?* 6. *How can cloud platforms improve data collaboration across healthcare institutions?*	Develop compliance-aware cloud architectures (e.g., HIPAA/GDPR-ready) Leverage edge-cloud hybrid models for real-time processing Conduct risk-benefit analysis of cloud migration in healthcare

As shown in Table 3.2, additional six research questions and possible approaches have been formulated to support the digital transformation of mission-related, management, and support operations in health management. These elements address research gaps that complement those discussed earlier.

3.2 PURSUING INNOVATION THROUGH HCRs AND EMRs IN HEALTHCARE

As part of meaningful use incentive, physicians and healthcare organizations were required to use EHRs/EMRs to take advantage of the $18B stimulus package for healthcare IT that was approved by the US congress in 2009.

As a result of the implementation of EHRs/EMRs in the last decade, a huge amount of data became available that allow healthcare organizations to take advantage of the data analytics for better decisions making. Even though EHRs/EMRs are used, doctors still prefer to use written-hand notes to update patient's records that are scanned and stored electronically as an image or a pdf format. That directs to searching the scanned records manually to find information needed about patents, which is a time consuming. This leads to inaccurate results because of human limited abilities the need of using big data in an innovation way appeared to be a worthy effort to develop a search methodology using technology and automations.

Healthcare organization seeks the ability to process data analytics from historical clinical records and notes to propose predictive risk or indicate KPIs in real-time, as seen in Figure 3.1. The accuracy of the information is essential to achieve financial advantage while competing with other healthcare organizations that serve the same patients. The proposed solution will help the leadership of the healthcare organizations to identify the weaknesses in their system that result in losing opportunities and market share, poor patient experience, and costly healthcare.

3.3 PRELIMINARY ARCHITECTURE FOR BIG DATA ANALYTICS

The performance indicators that the framework is going to provide as outcomes would focus on the operation services of the healthcare organization in the area of patient experience as demanded by the Center for Medicare and Medicaid Services' (CMS) quality guideline requirements. The framework should be capable to bring the optimization of processes workflow utilizing big data analytics to automate and customize the outcomes to align the performance indicators with the operation services of healthcare organization that need to be reported.

The framework shown in Figure 3.2 illustrates the conceptual idea of the model with separating the system in different layers as follows:

1. **The data source layer**.
2. **The data storage layer**: a repository data disk space to collect all data with different format types in one storage area.
3. **The data preparation layer**: responsible to segregate data with its own type.

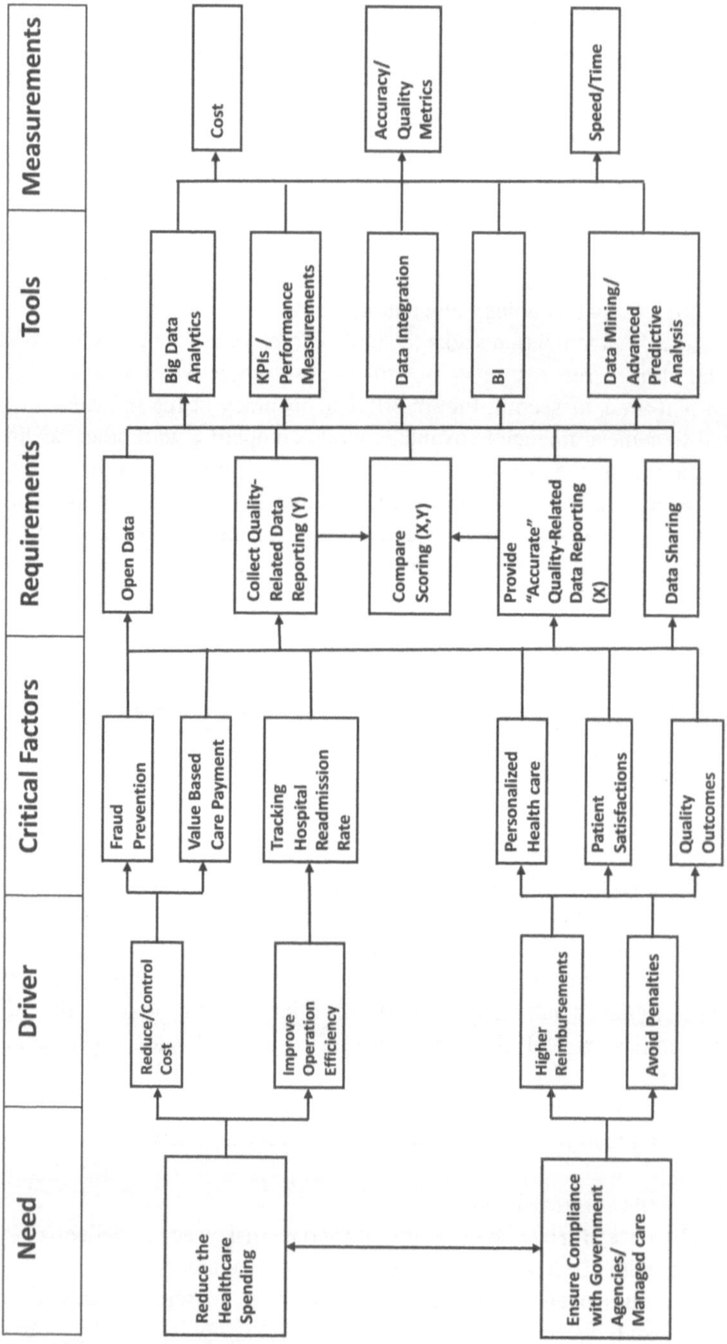

FIGURE 3.1 Smart relationship diagram.

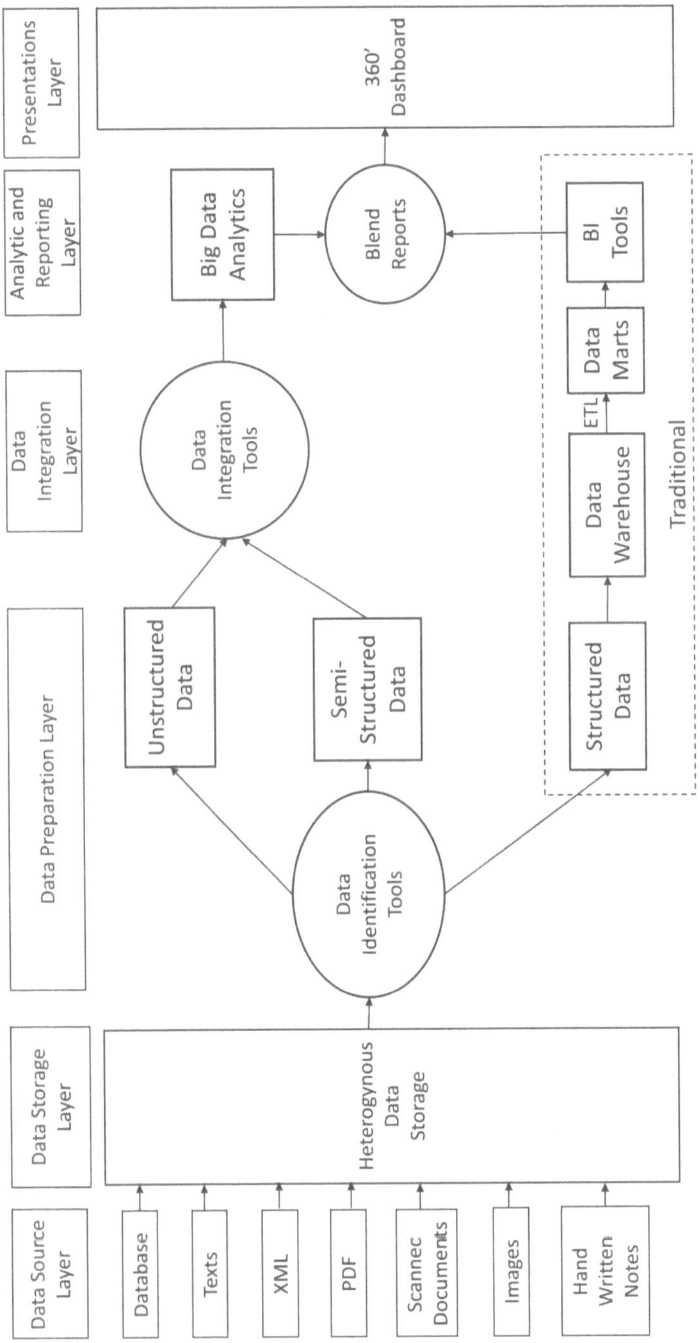

FIGURE 3.2 Big data analytics architecture.

4. **The data integration layer**: allows the consolidation and transformation between unstructured and semi-structured data types.
5. **The analytics and reporting layer**: provides operation reports and data analysis.
6. **The presentation layer**: visually shows KPIs and metrics.

3.4 CASE STUDY

The Center for Medicare and Medicaid Services (CMS) requires healthcare providers to submit an annual quality report for merit reimbursement as instructed in the Physician Quality Reporting System (PQRS) Program.

In the first week of January every year, the healthcare provider downloads a report from CMS portal that is saved in an excel file format. The report contains randomly selected patients who are treated at this healthcare provider through-out the year. This random sample of patients is picked from the total population of patients who are assigned to this healthcare provider by CMS. The report needs to be filled out with specific information according to CMS' metrics for this list of patients.

In 2017, CMS merged the PQRS program into the Merit-based Incentive Payment System (MIPS) and announced the change of the data submission method for 2018 report. The biggest change was that instead of entering a number that represented a specific value that met XML specifications (e.g., 1 = no, 2 = yes, etc.), they asked to select the appropriate answer from a dropdown box. CMS pushed out an excel template, which demonstrates this change and released the guide that explains the process.

The guidelines for 2019 have recently released and the case study will follow the new rules. The fact that CMS changes its rules every year, requires a fixable model that is easy to modify and adopt the new rules without revamping the existing model or creating a new system.

Generally, the metrics focus on measuring the following areas:

1. Diagnoses (Dx):
   a. Coronary artery disease (CAD)
   b. Diabetes
   c. Heart failure (HF)
   d. High blood pressure/Hypertension
   e. In vitro diagnostic (IVD): Use of aspirin or another antithrombotic
   f. Depression remission at 12 months

2. Ages:
   a. For patients with age between 50 and 75 years old: Colorectal cancer screening
   b. For women patients with age between 50 and 74 years old: Breast cancer screening
   c. For patients with 65 years old and older: Fall screening and pneumonia vaccination
   d. For patients with 18 years old and older:
      i. Document current meds,
      ii. BMI screening and follow-up plan,
      iii. Tobacco use: Screening and cessation intervention
      iv. Screen for high BP and follow-up plan.
   e. For patients with 12 years old and older: Screen for clinical depression and follow-up plan
   f. For patients with 6 months old and older: Influenza immunization
3. Age and diagnoses both combined:
   a. Statin therapy for the prevention and treatment of cardiovascular disease for ages:
      i. For patients older than 21 years old, previously diagnosed with arteriosclerotic cardiovascular disease (ASCVD)
      ii. For patients older than 21 years old, previous fasting/direct low-density-lipoprotein cholesterol—LDL-C ≥ 190 mg/dl
      iii. For patients between the age of 40 and 75 years old with Dx of Type 1 or 2 diabetes fasting/direct LDL-C level of 70–189 mg/dL

Currently, the information is obtained by manually searching tens of thousands of structured, semi-structured, and unstructured documents in a short period of time every year between the month of January and March. These documents contain an average of 4–5 pages that make hundreds of thousands of pages. This involves several workers to go through the pages via eye scan and manually looking for words/keywords based on metrics that CMS provided. After filling out the report with Yes/No on diagnosis and treatment, the provider submits the report before the deadline in the second or third week of March in the same year. CMS grades the report on accuracy for Continuum of Care and compare it against other providers on service for benchmarking of their performance measurements. If patient not accurately diagnosed with treatment, CMS would claw back bonus, merits, or change percentage of reimbursement. Therefore, this report is very essential for providers in their revenue income.

The health provider gets the information from its EHR care system that contains encrypted text notes (unstructured) and links to scanned images that

TABLE 3.3 CMS patient record verification and reporting process

STEP	*DESCRIPTION*
1	CMS has records of Medicare patients assigned or treated by each medical provider during the calendar year.
2	CMS selects a random sample from these records and assigns a unique ID for each patient.
3	CMS releases the list of patients in XML format to each provider's portal.
4	Healthcare provider downloads the list, converts it to Excel, and maps each CMS unique patient ID to their EHR system's patient ID.
5	Verify the status of each patient in the list:
5a	If *not found*, the patient is *ignored*.
5b	If *not qualified*, the provider explains the reason in the report.
6	For valid patients, perform eye scan, manual search, and analyze patient records according to CMS metric requests.
7	Fill in the list with information from EHR records, formatted according to CMS XML specifications.
8	Submit the completed file electronically via CMS portal before the deadline.
9	CMS compares the submitted data with data from other healthcare providers.
10	CMS benchmarks the performance of healthcare providers and adjusts merit and payment levels accordingly.

are stored outside the EHR database. This case study will answer if this process can be automated and would leveraging big data help? Table 3.3 shows the flow of events for the CMS Patient Record Verification and Reporting, and the CMS Patient Information Processing Workflow is presented in Table 3.4.

TABLE 3.4 CMS patient information processing workflow

STEP	*DESCRIPTION*
1	Access the EHR/EMR system and notes to extract information and documentation of patients listed by CMS.
2	Analyze each patient against CMS Metrics.
3	Send outputs of each patient in an Excel format file.
4	Consolidate all individual Excel files into one master file.
5	Save the consolidated Excel file according to CMS XML specifications.
6	Submit the completed file with the requested information electronically via the CMS portal.

3.5 VALIDATION AND LESSONS LEARNED

The validation of the model will be reached by comparing the outcomes of the model with the results out of the manual process. However, the functionality of the model will be tested operationally as a proof of concept (PoC), then the accuracy will be verified to ensure that the outputs have the desired quality of information. Additionally, the performance of the solution will be measured to reflect the speed and the time consumed to provide the requested information with comparison of achieving the same task manually.

3.6 FUTURE RESEARCH

The future research of big data in healthcare will focus toward building solutions that integrate all components of big data sources in visualization and cloud computing environments. Other areas of research will be conducted in mHealth, wearable devices, and IoT to improve the monitoring capabilities that provide quality healthcare to patients. This research will allow personalized treatment and real-time tracking of physical activities. Moreover, the needs for patients and providers to access the health records from anywhere via smart devices will lead researchers to introduce a standard protocol to access data universally in a better virtual and an infrastructure-less environment. Cloud computing and data analytics will be good areas of research that converts the clinical informatics into knowledge for better quality of healthcare. Innovative research in security will be needed to protect privacy when knowledge as a service (KaaS) is offered in large scale.

3.7 CONCLUSION

The ability of the framework to answer many of the questions in utilizing big data in healthcare performance measurements is clearly realized. It provided a better understanding of the impacts that big data is introducing in the financial, legal, and technology aspects. There are unlimited opportunities to improve the healthcare system utilizing health information technology and big data tools. It is still in its early stages of implementation but the employing of information technology in the medical field will stop the healthcare of holding up behind the rest of US economy. However, it is expected to happen as it did like other industries that had challenges. Healthcare systems, clinical practices, US government agencies, and insurance companies are all going to benefit from sharing the big data analytic for better quality of healthcare and the reduction per capita costs as well as good services to the community that they serve. Big data and predictive analytics are going to change the way healthcare organizations make decisions in both business and clinical areas, which should lead to reduce the economic risk.

Big data in healthcare introduces issues in patient information privacy that need to be addressed by the US government to regulate and organize sharing data. It is critical for healthcare organization to look at the big data and cloud computing from the perspective of management and marketing points of view to gain values of the long-term commitments.

REFERENCES

Aqeel, I., Khormi, I. M., Khan, S. B., Shuaib, M., Almusharraf, A., Alam, S., & Alkhaldi, N. A. (2023). Load balancing using artificial intelligence for cloud-enabled internet of everything in healthcare domain. *Sensors*, *23*(11). https://doi.org/10.3390/s23115349

Asri, H., & Jarir, Z. (2023). Toward a smart health: Big data analytics and IoT for real-time miscarriage prediction. *Journal of Big Data*, *10*(1), 34. https://doi.org/10.1186/s40537-023-00704-9

Awotunde, J. B., Panigrahi, R., Shukla, S., Panda, B., & Bhoi, A. K. (2024). Big data analytics enabled deep convolutional neural network for the diagnosis of cancer. *Knowledge and Information Systems*, *66*(2), 905–931. https://doi.org/10.1007/s10115-023-01971-x

Benzidia, S., Bentahar, O., Husson, J., & Makaoui, N. (2024). Big data analytics capability in healthcare operations and supply chain management: The role of green process innovation. *Annals of Operations Research*, *333*(2), 1077–1101. https://doi.org/10.1007/s10479-022-05157-6

Chatterjee, S., Chaudhuri, R., Gupta, S., Mangla, S. K., & Kamble, S. (2023). Examining the influence of industry 4.0 in healthcare supply chain performance: Moderating role of environmental dynamism. *Journal of Cleaner Production*, *427*, 139195. https://doi.org/10.1016/j.jclepro.2023.139195

Cho, M., Song, M., Park, J., Yeom, S.-R., Wang, I.-J., & Choi, B.-K. (2020). Process mining-supported emergency room process performance indicators. In *International Journal of Environmental Research and Public Health*, *17*(17). https://doi.org/10.3390/ijerph17176290

Demirbaga, U., & Aujla, G. S. (2022). MapChain: A blockchain-based verifiable healthcare service management in IoT-based big data ecosystem. *IEEE*

Transactions on Network and Service Management, *19*(4), 3896–3907. https://doi.org/10.1109/TNSM.2022.3204851

Fancy, C., Krishnaraj, N., Ishwarya, K., Raja, G., & Chandrasekaran, S. (2025). Modelling of healthcare data analytics using optimal machine learning model in big data environment. *Expert Systems*, *42*(1), e13612. https://doi.org/10.1111/exsy.13612

Hadi, M. S., Lawey, A. Q., El-Gorashi, T. E. H., & Elmirghani, J. M. H. (2020). Patient-centric HetNets powered by machine learning and big data analytics for 6g networks. *IEEE Access*, *8*, 85639–85655. https://doi.org/10.1109/ACCESS.2020.2992555

Hoque, A. S. M. L., Mia, M. R., Abdullah, M. S., Islam, M. J., Nath, B. C. D., Rahman, M. T., & Ahamed, S. I. (2024). BlockPRLS: Blockchain-Based Patient Record Linkage System for Big Data Analytics. *2024 IEEE 48th Annual Computers, Software, and Applications Conference (COMPSAC)*, 877–886. https://doi.org/10.1109/compsac61105.2024.00121

Jan, M. A., Zhang, W., Akbar, A., Song, H., Khan, R., & Chelloug, S. A. (2024). A hybrid mutual authentication approach for artificial intelligence of medical things. *IEEE Internet of Things Journal*, *11*(1), 311–320. https://doi.org/10.1109/JIOT.2023.3317292

Korayim, D., Chotia, V., Jain, G., Hassan, S., & Paolone, F. (2024). How big data analytics can create competitive advantage in high-stake decision forecasting? the mediating role of organizational innovation. *Technological Forecasting and Social Change*, *199*, 123040. https://doi.org/10.1016/j.techfore.2023.123040

Kumar, R. H., & Sunitha, G. (2024). Big data analytics in healthcare environment using chaotic red deer optimizer with deep learning for disease classification model. *Multimedia Tools and Applications*, *83*(32), 77697–77715. https://doi.org/10.1007/s11042-024-18239-3

Ristevski, B., & Chen, M. (2018). Big data analytics in medicine and healthcare. *Journal of Integrative Bioinformatics*, 15(3), 20170030. https://doi.org/10.1515/jib-2017-0030

Scorza, A., Porazzi, E., Strozzi, F., Garagiola, E., Gimigliano, A., & De Filippis, G. (2022). A new approach for emergency department performance positioning: The quality-efficiency matrix. *The International Journal of Health Planning and Management*, *37*(3), 1636–1649. https://doi.org/10.1002/hpm.3428

Wang, Y., Kung, L., & Byrd, T. A. (2018). Big data analytics: Understanding its capabilities and potential benefits for healthcare organizations. *Technological Forecasting and Social Change*, *126*, 3–13. https://doi.org/10.1016/j.techfore.2015.12.019

Yu, W., Zhao, G., Liu, Q., & Song, Y. (2021). Role of big data analytics capability in developing integrated hospital supply chains and operational flexibility: An organizational information processing theory perspective. *Technological Forecasting and Social Change*, *163*, 120417. https://doi.org/10.1016/j.techfore.2020.120417

Research Framework 4

The key to leading successful big data analytics for healthcare organizations (HCOs) is establishing a framework in an actionable approach with descriptive structure that complies with their strategic imperatives and digital capabilities to become a data analytics-driven HCO that leads to the improvement of the performance of clinical, financial, and operational outcomes. The objective of the framework is to extend the HCO's data ecosystem in an innovative way that leverages emerging technologies such as big data and offers the integration of technological platforms and advanced analytics.

The goal of the study is to assess the framework by measuring the desired outcomes to HCOs using big data analytics.

4.1 PROPOSED FRAMEWORK

Developing a framework of big data analytics for healthcare enterprises incorporates the people, process, and technology models as a good foundation to add on top of another three elements: organization, the data, and the outcomes. The relationship of all six components of the frameworks would lead to automation, standardization, and innovation for successful outcomes.

People is defined as all the stakeholders such as leaderships, employees, and customers, who are involved in turning medical information into value that serves clients and meets their needs. Processes incorporate the actions to employ the organization's strategy for delivering needed services for customers and to automate processes when it is possible. Technology entails the ability to use computers and applications to collect and save data from customers for analyzing, in order to improve better outcomes to customer needs with accurate information in real time (Almotairi, 2009).

The proposed framework includes the source of data, data governance and processes, data life cycle, defining metrics/key performance indicators

DOI: 10.1201/9781003610731-4

(KPIs), and determining the criteria for selecting the proper analytics tools. Furthermore, the framework contains information about the appropriate infrastructure for hosting in the cloud or on-premises. Identifying skill sets and resources is also part of the proposed framework.

Additionally, Cates et al. (2005) showed the amalgamation of people, process, and technology in their model of "The Ladder of Business Intelligence (LOBI)" that presented six levels of maturity: facts, data, information, knowledge, understanding, and enabled intuition. Thus, the framework aims to reach the level of enabled intuition by using the data completeness to provide directions to HCOs' future state to mature their data usage and enhance their existing capabilities.

To fully realize the capabilities of big data, implementing a tool to analyze data is not sufficient; a framework that blends people, processes, and technology is necessary to achieve value. Technical people with the right skills, knowledge, and competencies are key elements in the framework. Managing data that addresses how to govern the data and its lifecycle is an important component in controlling the domains in which HCOs have a wide range of available data. From a technological perspective, it is about tools, platforms, and technology infrastructure. Therefore, the right framework is not data or technology centric. Still, it should be an adequate combination of these components where, if it is implemented, it allows HCOs to have the ability to innovate in a sustainable way, help them to target specific opportunities, and drive their strategic imperatives.

The framework is to connect all components together and to offer a simple landscape that is more powerful and adds value to take advantage of big data capabilities, 3Vs as an example.

The most powerful advances of the framework are the emphasis in patient care and receiving data in real-time in a centralized location, without separating forms of data as these are considered data capture vehicles as well as data delivery vehicles, whether it's off an EMR entry, a wearable patient device, telehealth, or a patient monitoring data that are all considered sources of big data which, we use to do analytics against and extract knowledge in real time to the clinical and business areas.

Additionally, the framework needs to ensure the inclusiveness of the data from all areas and data quality through assurance mechanisms to give the organization a level of confidence and trust of the coming outputs of metric and KPI. Therefore, having data governance that defines data ownership and deals with the accuracy of the data and when it will be obsolete is an essential element in the framework.

The proposed framework shown in Figure 4.1 includes 41 essential entities categorized in 6 different areas: Organization, people, processes, data, technology, and outcomes.

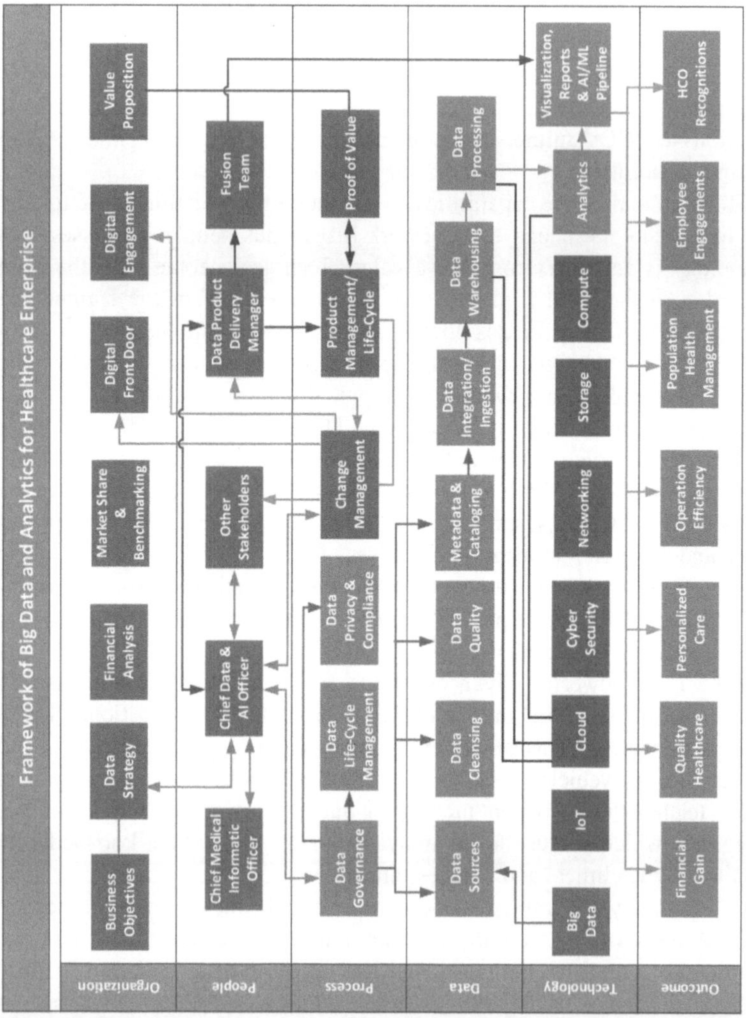

FIGURE 4.1 Proposed big data and analytics framework for healthcare enterprise.

Each entity represents a function, or a role and some entities are linked to one or more entities. The standalone entities that are not linked to any others are still crucial to the framework for a complete view.

The linked entities are connected with a straight line to show their linkage. The one-way or two-way arrow indicates that there is an interaction between the two entities in one direction or in both directions. Additionally, the line with the direction of the arrow implies a relationship between several entities that interact together in several but similar channels.

The blocks display the entities in groups to construct a cluster for a distinct purpose. The big data entity is the main component in the framework, and it is under the technology area. The framework's core places all data and analytics entities in one group, distributed among processes, data, and technology areas. Other blocks show the technologies that are needed to utilize big data and analytics. Some blocks are the supportive entities in the framework that guarantee a successful result. The outcome blocks show the expected value of adopting big data analytics. The proposed framework is refined, and each entity encompasses much work and resources.

4.1.1 Healthcare System and Data Mapping

It is important to understand the healthcare industry to construct the appropriate framework that directs the priorities and ventures of the HCO to reach its goals. There are several departments in healthcare that are required to interact with each other to present the organization as a healthcare system.

The mapping of the healthcare system in Figure 4.2 illustrates the relationship of the necessary segments of the framework and their involvements in big data and analytics. At the organization level, the vision and the strategy are built around the patients. Not only to provide the needed care during illness but also to keep them healthy. All departments in the healthcare system exist to serve patients in the clinical setting or in the business side. Many departments such as supply chain and information technology do not interact directly with patients, but they are crucial in the daily operations. Data and technology are utilized for creating metrics that are available for internal and external users.

4.1.1.1 Healthcare business

The modularity of the healthcare system and the orchestration among departments cannot be achieved without a strong ecosystem that supplies intuition of real time activities. It starts with the leadership team for laying the organization strategy by outlining the goals, the vision, and the value as well

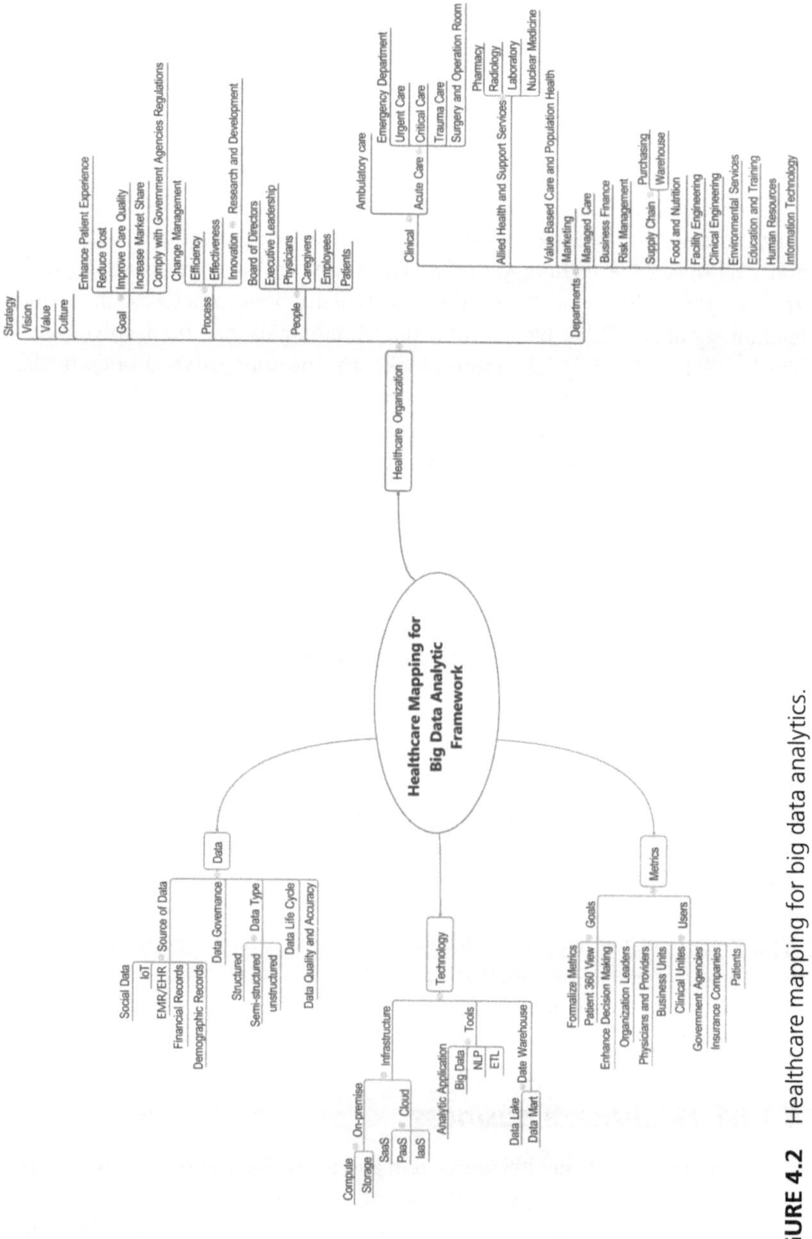

FIGURE 4.2 Healthcare mapping for big data analytics.

as planning, analyzing the market, and setting performance measurement targets.

As a result of the fourth Industrial Revolution (I4.0), healthcare is moving toward a new paradigm with Healthcare 4.0 (H4.0), where healthcare business shifts from hospital-centered to patient-care focus (Tortorella et al., 2020).

Everything patient-related should be at the core of the strategy, employing technologies to enhance capabilities in its ecosystem. The organization's vision must endorse digitalization to benefit from all available analyzed data and be willing to invest significant capital and operational funds to deliver an excellent digital experience to data consumers such as clinicians, business units, and patients.

Therefore, data analytics should be one of the top strategic imperatives that the organization's leadership wants to attain. The business objectives of adopting big data analytics must be communicated clearly to stakeholders to ensure they stand behind this objective. The organization's value will be realized when data innovation is embraced. Neglecting it could cause the organization to lose market share and revenue. Thus, data analytics is a linchpin to other emerging technologies such as AI/ML. When the data project is approved, listing the project goals is required to reference the organization's strategy to assure alignment. Securing funds and resources, defining the scope, and creating the project schedule are parts of the project planning. Measuring the project performance in meeting the scope, finance and timeframe is essential for discernibility.

Additionally, a key success factor is the need to design processes to receive or provide data to and from departments within or with other healthcare systems. Process design is the center of the overall roadmap to transform the organization into a data-driven organization. It concentrates on the goals based on the organization's purpose, vision, and values that are defined at the organization level. Process planning should align with strategic planning to translate it into a tangible task when the data project starts. Measurable means should be identified at the organization, process, and data project levels to evaluate the success of the desired outcomes. At the organizational level, the balanced scorecard (BSC) is a measurable means of achieving financial and operational goals. KPI is another measurable method that validates the success of reaching business goals. At the process level, the aim is to measure the process capability (C_{PK}/P_{PK}) that determines whether the specifications are met.

The healthcare business is required to revamp its processes around the new capability that digital transformation introduced to the industry for greater effectiveness and efficiency. The revised processes should describe how each department will deal with the data it generates or uses and how it

TABLE 4.1 Mapping organization, process and data project

LEVEL	*GOALS*	*DESIGN*	*MEASUREMENT*
Organization	Purpose/Vision/Value	Strategic plan	BSC/KPI
Process	Process goals	Process design	C_{PK}/P_{PK}
Data project	Project goals	Project plan	Project performance

will be shared with other departments within the same organization and/or other HCOs.

Table 4.1 shows the mapping of organization, process, and data projects and how they relate to the goals, design, and measurement.

The Information Technology (IT) department is the main player that implements the infrastructure and applications and is responsible for controlling and securing data access. IT is expected to rapidly respond to business and regulatory obligations with technical solutions and products.

The Communications and Marketing departments can use the data to discover how the community that the HCO serves feels and how they can gain their trust. Indeed, social media is one element that needs close attention to capitalize on the positive comments of patient real-time feedback and focus on correcting any negative remarks.

The Regulatory, Public Affairs, and Government Relations departments interface with politicians and state governments, which set legal rules and laws regulating healthcare benefits for state citizens. Providing accurate data about the health of the community and patients is essential in establishing trust between the HCO and local and state governments.

The Human Resources (HR) department needs to collaborate with other departments to fill the number of employees needed. Insight from data analytics allows planning to adjust the number of employees for each shift by hiring more or reassigning them to areas that are short-staffed.

Having data is also a liability. The Legal department is expected to provide guidance to avoid lawsuits against the HCO. They establish guidelines for the policies and procedures required by the law. They must also know the impact of digitalization on legal counseling when using or sharing data on patients' health.

The Audit and Compliance department can employ data analytics in audits and fraud Prevention. They should work with IT Security to develop policies and procedures to track the access of patients' health information to prevent misuse of the data or sharing with other entities that may result in legal actions.

Business finance and budget fund projects and initiatives. They control the spending of money. Therefore, their involvement is crucial to secure the necessary capital for the data analytics initiatives. They also use the outcomes of data analytics to forecast the financial plan for fiscal years based on growth and market share. The Account Payable department can gain value out of big data as many invoices are scanned as images and need manual labor for verification and auditing.

Supply Chain is another department that can benefit from big data in many forms. In the area of warehousing and inventory, using IoT technology allows locating parts and supplies in a very effective way, and it accurately provides the available inventories so that no shortage or overstocking of medical supplies or medications occur.

Revenue Management is the account receivable that is in charge for the process of invoicing patients to their medical billing. Big data that includes unstructured and semi-structured data to the analytics can improve the financial results and increase revenue. It can help in analyzing market access, foresee readmission and benchmarking of efficiency and comparative analysis.

The Care Management department deals with insurance claims for reimbursements. Big data analytics simplifies the process of providing quality reports to Medicare and Medicate government agencies as well as preventing insurance frauds.

Clinical Engineering and Facility Engineering departments that support the medical equipment and buildings can monitor devices and perform predictive maintenance utilizing IoT technology that reports alarms from equipment malfunctions and issues with the temperature of drugs refrigerators.

Finally, care delivery is the main beneficiary of big data analytics, which helps deliver quality care to patients in many aspects. One area is pattern recognition in image processing of MRI, X-ray, and ultrasound using deep learning to discover abnormalities. Additionally, many HCOs participate in clinical research in areas such as genetics, genomics, and precision medicine for drug development and innovations.

4.1.1.2 Stakeholders

The goal of identifying stakeholder is to assess and comprehend their significance, interactions, impacts, authority, and interests toward a successful initiative (Brugha & Varvasovszky, 2000).

Several stakeholders are involved in the data analytics process. The main stakeholders are the individuals or entities who provide the data, analyze the data, and receive the outcomes of the data analytics. The leaders of the HCO are consumers of the data analytics outcomes that allow them to determine their organization's performance and understand market shares to engender business value.

The Chief Medical Officer (CMO), Chief Quality Officer—Medicine (CQO-M), and Chief Nursing Officer (CNO) are the clinical leaders who should be consulted on achieving the desired outcomes of using the data and involved in the data strategic imperative.

The Chief Financial Officer (CFO), Chief Operating Officer (COO), Chief Revenue Officer (CRO), and Chief Compliance and ethics Officer are the business leaders who also need to be included in the discussion of the data strategy to provide input on the data they can provide and the reports they desire.

Healthcare Regulatory Agencies are external stakeholders such as the Centers for Medicare & Medicaid Services (CMS), the Agency for Health Care Administration (AHCA), that demand specific reports and conduct inspections to certify the HCO's processes, quality, and facilities to practice as healthcare providers. In addition, managed care and insurance companies request quality reports from their customers to whom they provide health insurance.

The data professional team consists of several groups, and it is supervised by the Chief Data and AI Officer (CDAIO), whose main objective is to lead the HCO to use data and emerging technology in analytics to produce value by enhancing clinical delivery and improving business performance. CDAIO guides the HCO in its data strategy to incorporate digitalization and innovation to widen its ability to leverage data analytics to expand its ecosystem. The role of the CDAIO is to bridge data and business together to guarantee alignment of goals and identify opportunities. Furthermore, CDAIO establishes communication channels with leadership and physicians to transform the organization's culture to value data by educating and sharing information. Additionally, CDAIO drives the relationship with technology vendors and partners to select the appropriate technology platforms and software tools for data analytics and endorses following best practices when implemented. Moreover, CDAIO conducts a cross-functional data governance to attain data control and quality for accurate outcomes. Identifying the needed roles of data professionals is one of the essential jobs of CDAIO, helping them develop their skillsets in the data era. The data professional teams include the data engineers, whose main tasks are coding, developing, and verifying data quality end-to-end. The data scientists' task is to build algorithm models and use statistics to boost outcomes by extracting useful information from raw data. The Data Business Analysis team analyzes data reported from customers, business, and cross-departmental. They work with the business relationship management team to ensure that data is collected and analyzed according to business demands. Additionally, the data integration team's main function is to allow data sharing among systems.

Technology vendors and partners are identified as external stakeholders, and their support in accomplishing the goals of the data strategy is critical.

They are at the core of the framework in both the financial and technology aspects.

Clinicians, providers, physicians, and caregivers are the major suppliers who enter patients' health information data into the EMR/EHR systems and use the results of the analyzed data to make medical decisions and/or conduct medical research.

Finally, HCOs target patients by delivering quality healthcare and allowing patients easy access to their health information, as well as making appointments and paying their bills.

4.1.1.3 Process mapping

Process mapping is a way to embody the procedures of the business in a visual technique to assist in comprehending the steps of the process. The purpose of process mapping is to evaluate and clarify to improve the process and the ability to measure each action in the process (Klotz et al., 2008).

Process mapping is an essential stage in creating the framework as it does layout the steps of the patient journey from start to finish. It shows the patient's involvement from the time treatment begins until the service of care is fully paid and how the sequence of activities of each department is involved during the treatment (Trebble et al., 2010).

Comprehensive Health Record (CHR) is the evolution of EHR/EMR, which the leaders of the patient electronic records software development companies prefer to use as a new term instead of EHR/EMR. In addition to the medical and health records, CHR also includes essential collected data beyond the healthcare provider settings, such as social determinants and behavioral care (Sullivan, 2017). Thus, the CHR term is used in the process mapping.

The process mapping for outpatients, emergency department (ED) patients, and inpatients has several workstreams with similar steps. The types of data collected during the scheduling and check-in/registration steps entail patient accounting, demographics, and insurance information. During treatment, medical records, diagnoses, and/or procedure codes are entered for each patient encounter, as well as medical order entries and results.

Moreover, revenue cycle management and external data also contribute to the data the system gathers or uses. Data about payments, billing, bad debt, and collections is identified in the system as part of the revenue cycle management. External data from social media or produced by IoT and monitoring devices is also reflected in the process mapping as part of the data sources.

The healthcare process mapping in Figure 4.3 illustrates the relationship of all entities in the healthcare system and their involvement in generating big data that is being analyzed.

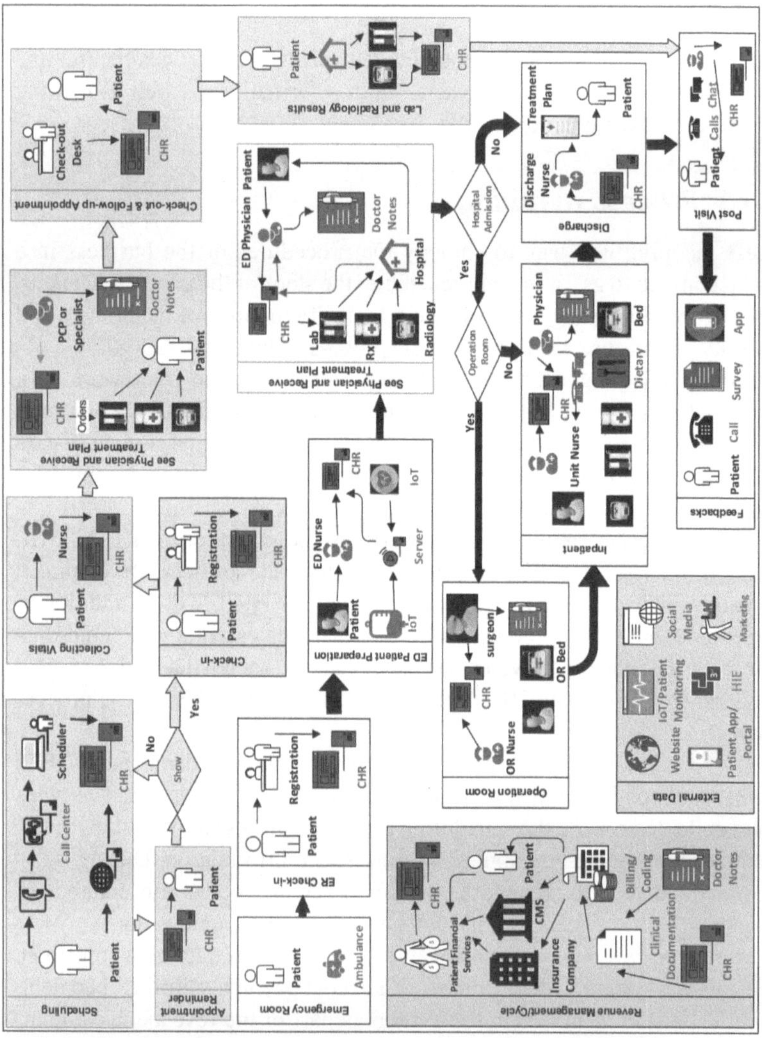

FIGURE 4.3 Process map of data creation in healthcare.

4.1.1.4 SIPOC-R

Suppliers, inputs, processes, outputs, customers, and requirements (SIPOC-R) is a quality tool that aids in understanding the elements of a process and its requirements (Sarkar et al., 2011). The process is the flow of actions that list the "HOWs", the inputs and outputs describe the WHATs, and the suppliers and customers identify the WHOs (Parkash & Kaushik, 2011).

Understanding the demands of the suppliers and customers is essential for knowing how the data is gathered and stored. Thus, SIPOC-R makes the digital journey of a patient easy to understand by identifying the suppliers and the data customers involved in each step of the process. Moreover, the inputs and the outputs of each step of the process determine the submitted information by the suppliers and the data delivered to the customers. Requirements determine the needs of each step for a successful execution.

The SIPOC-R of data created for outpatients begins with scheduling appointments to see a physician or a medical service, such as lab work or radiology. Recording the call is considered unstructured data that needs to be analyzed to evaluate customer satisfaction with the overall service. The patient or the guarantor provides the needed information, mostly structured data, whether he/she is a new or an existing patient, to the scheduler or via an online application. Before the visit, the system reaches out to the patient for an appointment reminder and asks to confirm, cancel, or reschedule the appointment. On the day of the visit, the patient's information is verified and updated during the check-in process or flagged as a no-show if the patient does not show up. The show/no-show status is another data point that can help the business adjust the overbooking ratio. Additionally, knowing the cause of no-shows can allow the HC system to help patients who need transportation. Measuring the waiting time before the patient enters the examination room is another data that can be easily collected to enhance the patient experience.

In fact, the system can measure each step's time in the evaluation and enhancement process. The nurse collects the vitals in the examination room and enters them into the CHR system. The most important data that most likely was not entered into the system is the conversation between the physician and the patient, usually documented in handwritten notes. This unstructured data is the main challenge for many HCOs as it is missing in the claims submitted to payers or CMS for payments. In this situation, SIPOC-R tools help recognize this data and its location in the system. Physicians also enter the diagnosis code in the CHR system as structured data. When patients check out, they get the discharged paperwork with subscribed work orders for lab or radiology. They can also schedule a follow-up for a future appointment, if needed.

When performed outside the HCOs, lab results and radiology reports cannot be included in the CHR and will be missed in the submitted claims. Therefore, a post-visit follow-up call with the patient is needed to ensure the directions from the physician are pursued. It is also a good opportunity to hear the patient's feedback of their experience during the visit. The follow-up call can be recorded and analyzed as part of big data analytics. Table 4.2 shows the SIPOC-R of data generated for outpatients.

Similarly, the SIPOC-R of data for ED has a minor modification as it does not need prior scheduled appointment and it can lead to admission as inpatient or for a surgery. Additionally, the IoT and the monitoring devices hooked to the patient feed the system with semi and unstructured data. Also, all the lab work and radiology orders performed internally and external data using HIE from external sources can be reviewed for patient health history. The discharge process is more sophisticated than the outpatient process because HCOs could be penalized if the patient is discharged prematurely and is readmitted for the same illness within a short period from his/her first admission. Table 4.3 shows the SIPOC-R of creating data for ED patients.

For inpatients, the SIPOC-R is a combination of outpatient and inpatient SIPOC-Rs, except that surgery is needed. Patients are admitted to the hospital with a physician order, scheduled surgery, or from the ED. Table 4.4 shows the SIPOC-R of data for inpatient.

Revenue cycle management is the most critical department in the HCOs, and it is considered the main consumer of the generated data in the form of clinical documentation that brings income to the organization via submitting claims to CMS and health insurance payers. In addition to unstructured data of handwritten notes and the structured data entry to the CHR system, specialists, and care givers use dictation using voice recognition software to describe the diagnoses of the case and the protocol used for treatment. Then a medical transcriptionist listens to the recorded voice and updates the written report accordingly. This process can be automated using big data analytics as the voice recordings and the written reports are considered semi-structured and unstructured data. The clinical report is part of the clinical documentation that is needed for claim submissions, and it must be accurate to avoid denying the claim. It also needs to be complete with the correct treatment codes for proper payments. Moreover, the information included in the clinical documentation contributes to the quality reports submitted to payers and government agencies as illustrated in the causal loop diagram (CLD) of data and quality section. Patient financial services prepare invoices to collect payments and enter data to the CHR system as appropriate.

Table 4.5 shows SIPOC-R of each step of creating or consuming data in for the revenue cycle management.

TABLE 4.2 SIPOC-R for outpatient data

CYCLE	*SUPPLIER*	*INPUT*	*PROCESS*	*OUTPUT*	*CUSTOMER*	*REQUIREMENTS*
1	Patient	Patient's demographics	Schedule an appointment	Appointment made	Scheduler	Call center CHR
2	System auto-call	Appointment information	Appointment reminder	Confirmation/ cancellation	Patient	Call center CHR
3	Patient	Patient's verification/co-pay	Patient check-in	Patient checked-in/ waiting	Registration/ check-in-desk	CHR
4	Patient	Vital signs/reason for visit	Collecting vitals	Vitals collected/ entered in CHR	Nurse	CHR
5	Patient	Patient explanation of sickness	Seeing PCP/ specialist	Diagnoses (ICD-10), Rx, lab, radiology, doctor notes	PCP/specialist	CHR, typing note, pen/paper
6	Nurse/ Check-out clerk	Treatment plan, schedule follow-up appointment	Check-out	Printout orders and follow up appointment	Patient	CHR and printers
7	Patient	Lab or radiology workorder	Lab and/or radiology order	Lab and radiology reports/results	Laboratory or radiology center	Lab/Radiology system. fax or integration interface
8	Nurse or physician	Follow-up with patient on results	Post visit	Status information and guidance	Patient	CHR, and call or secure chat

TABLE 4.3 SIPOC-R for ED patient data

CYCLE	*SUPPLIER*	*INPUT*	*PROCESS*	*OUTPUT*	*CUSTOMER*	*REQUIREMENTS*
1	Patient	Patient's demographics	Patient check-in	Patient checked-in/ waiting	Registration/ Check-in-desk	CHR
2	Patient	Vital signs/reason for visit	Collecting vitals/ patient ED ready	Vitals collected, entered in CHR, monitoring data	ED nurse	CHR/IoT monitoring
3	Patient	Patient explanation of pain	Seeing ED physician	Initial diagnoses, Rx, Lab, radiology orders, doctor notes	ED physician	CHR, typing note, pen/paper
4	Patient	Rx, lab, and/or radiology workorder	Fill out Rx, lab and/or radiology order	Workorder performed	ED Lab/ pharmacy/ radiology departments	CHR, Rx, lab/ radiology system
5	ED Lab/radiology departments	Rx, lab, and/or radiology	Sending results of lab/radiology workorders	Lab and radiology reports	ED physician	CHR
6	ED physician	Lab and radiology reports doctor notes	Diagnoses	Treatment plan doctor notes	Patient/ED nurse	CHR, typing note, pen/paper
7	ED discharge/ admission nurse	Treatment plan, schedule follow-up appointment	Discharge or admission	Printout orders and follow up with PCP/ specialist	Patient	CHR and printers
8	Nurse or physician	Follow-up with patient	Post visit	Status information and guidance	Patient	CHR, and call or secure chat

TABLE 4.4 SIPOC-R for inpatient data

CYCLE	*SUPPLIER*	*INPUT*	*PROCESS*	*OUTPUT*	*CUSTOMER*	*REQUIREMENTS*
1	Patient	Patient's demographics	Patient check-in	Patient checked-in/ waiting for room (or OR)	Registration/ check-in-desk	CHR
2	Patient	Vital signs/reason for visit	Collecting vitals/ make patient ready	Vitals collected, entered in CHR, monitoring data	Nurse	CHR/IoT monitoring
3	Patient	Patient explanation of admission	Seeing physician/ surgeon	Patient ready for treatment or surgery, doctor notes	Physician/ surgeon	CHR, typing note, pen/paper
4	Physician/ Surgeon	Treatment plan	Perform surgery	Surgery performed, surgery data and doctor notes	Patient	CHR, OR, Rx, lab/ radiology system
5	Unit nurse, physician(s)	Treatment plan, doctor notes	Illness treatment	Updated treatment plan, doctor notes	Patient	CHR, typing note, pen/paper
6	Physician	Lab and radiology reports, doctor notes	Pre-discharge	Doctor notes	Patient/ ED nurse	CHR, typing note, pen/paper
7	ED discharge nurse	Treatment plan, schedule follow-up appointment	Discharge	Printout orders and follow up with PCP/specialist	Patient	CHR and printers
8	Nurse or physician	Follow-up with patient	Post visit	Status information and guidance	Patient	CHR, and call or secure chat

TABLE 4.5 SIPOC-R for revenue cycle/management data

CYCLE	*SUPPLIER*	*INPUT*	*PROCESS*	*OUTPUT*	*CUSTOMER*	*REQUIREMENTS*
1	Physicians	Voice dictations	Voice recording to list diagnoses/ treatments	Voice recording	Voice recognition software	Voice recognition software
2	Voice recognition software	Voice recording	Converting physicians dictations to capture items for billing	Medical written report	Medical transcriptionist	CHR/Voice recognition software
3	CHR/Computer systems/ external health records	CHR, HIE, doctor notes, medical reports	Organizing, reviewing medical records with correct billing code	Clinical documentation with captured coded items for billing	Clinical documentation specialist	CHR, HIE, written note, medical reports, clinical documentation system
4	Clinical documentation specialist	Clinical documentation with captured coded items for billing	Billing preparation	Surgery performed, surgery data and doctor notes	Patient financial services	CHR, clinical documentation system
5	Patient financial services	Treatment plan, doctor notes	Submitting claim to payers	Claim sent	Insurance company/CMS	CHR, mail, electronic data transfer
6	Patient financial services	Billing statement	Collecting payments	Billing statement sent	Patient	CHR, mail, calls
7	Patient/ insurance company/CMS	Send payment	Make payments	Payments received and updated account	Patient financial services	CHR

4.1.2 Data in Healthcare

Digital transformation in healthcare started when the American Recovery and Reinvestment Act (ARRA) demanded all HCOs and providers to fulfill meaningful use requirements by implementing electronic medical records (EMR) in 2014 to sustain their current eligibility for providing care to Medicaid and Medicare patients. It was followed by the Health Information Technology for Economic and Clinical Health Act (HITECH Act) to encourage HCOs to convert medical records from paper charts into digital forms by giving incentives when HCOs procure certified EMR/EHR systems and follow the guidelines of privacy regulations and accuracy. Before that time, data was scattered in different systems with one capability for a specific area and a labor-intensive process. EMR/EHR helped to integrate systems and eliminate the silos among them into one system. However, many physicians still use handwritten notes for their patients that cannot be entered into the EMT/EHR system as computerized data. Still, it is scanned and saved as an image, or they type note in a plain text format saved within the EMR/EHR system. Nevertheless, neither scanned nor plain text has a structured format that can be analyzed. Therefore, emerging technologies, such as big data technology, were needed to exploit unused data.

Adaptation of these new emerging technologies allowed linking events when triggered in one area to take actions in other areas which helped in eliminating the disconnect among departments.

The efforts of digitalization in healthcare took another milestone step when HCOs started to exchange patient information for better and faster care through health information exchange (HIE) within Region, State, or the United States. HIE enables HCOs to share and exchange patient records electronically by participating in Interorganizational Information System (IOIS) (Adjerid et al., 2018). The goals of creating HIE are to prevent readmissions, stop prescription drug errors, enhancing diagnoses, and reduces unnecessary replicate testing (*HealthIT.Gov Website*, n.d.).

4.1.2.1 Source of data in healthcare

Data completeness in healthcare comes from several sources and each system has its own data mart that makes the data ready for analytics. The primary source of data is the EMR/EHR system that contains demographic information about the patient such as home address, age, gender, race, etc.

It also contains blood pressure, height, and weight. The EMR/EHR system enters diagnoses of diseases based on ICD-9 and ICD-10 classification codes, medications, and lab results.

Another data source is enterprise resource planning (ERP), a system that consolidates business applications in one software suite and manages the functionality of the business in finance, accounting, HR, operations, and administrative tasks.

4.1.2.2 Big data and quality improvement relationship in healthcare

Quality metrics need data; the more data incorporated, the more insight. Quality 4.0 is the digitalization of traditional quality management, and big data is an essential element to improve the quality of design, the quality of service, and the quality of conformance (Sony et al., 2020). Therefore, many HCOs have started to explore big data analytics for comprehensive quality measurement.

Most healthcare providers and organizations lack technology and insufficient data to create performance measurement reports for government agencies for accreditations and payments linked to performance. Additionally, the performance reports are publicly published for transparency, and poor outcomes can cause a bad reputation that leads to a drop in market share and a decline in business (Nelson et al., 2005). Big data technology successfully addresses the challenge of inadequate data, allowing for good-quality reports. Mortality, readmission, patient experience, and efficiency and effectiveness in care are the performance measures that quality reports need to include. Big data is a key driver for delivering performance reports with high accuracy and complete information.

In 2016, CMS revealed the star rating program at the hospital level. Which is an easy-to-understand system that is based on the level of quality care, with a range of one star as the lowest rating to five stars as the highest rating, based on the hospital's performance of certain quality metrics (Hu & Nerenz, 2020).

At the provider practices level, CMS implemented the Medicare Shared Savings Program (MSSP) in 2012 as part of the Accountable Care Organization (ACO) model to promote collaboration among providers and specialists to share bonus reimbursement based on overall savings because of the superior quality care (Ouayogodé et al., 2017).

McCurdy (2001) enumerated HC Accreditation Organizations with increasing comparison of their accreditation programs and the target HC entities. The study indicated that the number of HCOs requesting accreditation is continually increasing to satisfy the requirements of the state and government agencies to maintain their care certification. It also illustrated the accreditation conditions of quality performance for accepting HCOs under their accreditation program umbrella. The National Committee on Quality Assurance (NCQA), Joint Commission on Accreditation of Healthcare Organizations (JCAHO), and the American Accreditation Healthcare Commission (URAC) are the three major accreditation institutes. All operate under not-for-profit organization status.

Other institutes offer high-performance awards to extraordinary HCOs for their high-quality achievements by being benchmarked and adopting innovations by using emerging data technologies during their digitalization transformation journey. HCOs receive awards by being ranked high by institutes such as IBM Watson Top 100 hospitals, Leapfrog grade, US News & World Report rankings, and HIMSS Most Wired, a prestigious recognition that positions them as exceptional leaders in the HC industry.

Emergency Care Research Institute (ECRI) is another independent, not-for-profit organization that serves as an evaluator of patient safety, evidence-based medicine, and technology decision support that leads to safer, more efficient, and higher effectiveness HC (*ECRI Website*, n.d.).

4.1.2.3 Causal loop diagram (CLD) of big data and quality

The dense and vigorous condition of the processes within the healthcare ecosystem, combined with the data life cycle, can lead to efforts to attain high-quality outcomes with the anticipation of increasing revenue and market share.

The CLD shown in Figure 4.4 exemplifies the relationship between data, quality, and profit in healthcare. More data provides extra perceptiveness that helps clinical and business sectors make better decisions. On the business side, it is a tangible method to control operating expenditure by avoiding overstaffing and projecting the appropriate number of workers based on needs. On the clinical side, incomplete patient data can cause delays in diagnosing illness and providing the right treatments promptly, which can likely alleviate the length of stay (LOS).

Data incompleteness is a pivotal challenge for HCOs when they submit quality reports to government agencies and insurance companies about patients they treat, resulting in a failure to get reimbursement. Therefore, technology such as big data is valuable in process automation, which can reduce the manual procedures and man-hours needed to create quality reports.

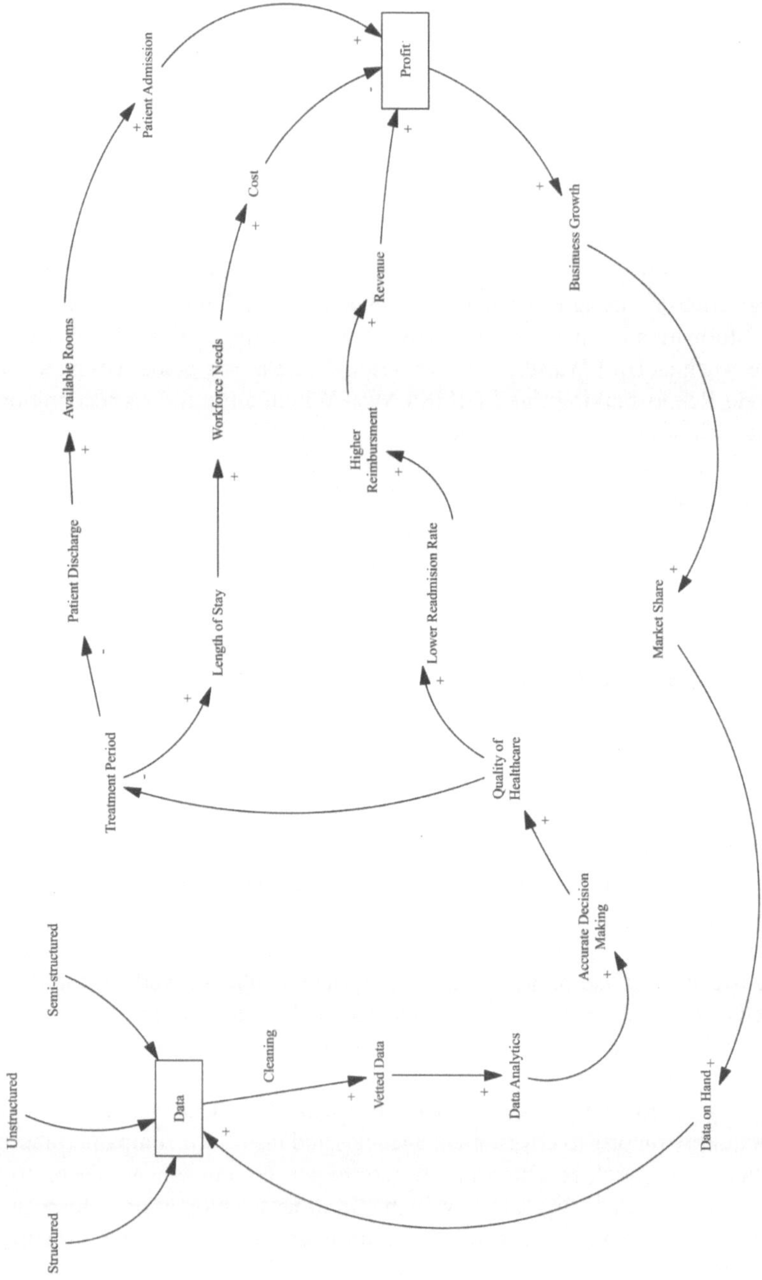

FIGURE 4.4 CLD data, quality, and profit.

4.1.3 Big Data Tools

Big data platform analytics is one of the foundational digital capabilities, whether it is systems or tools for improving outcomes. Commonly, many HCOs have numerous numbers of both embedded analytics and standalone analytics applications, many of which are duplicates as they were purchased in an ad-hoc fashion based on departmental needs. This approach would not scale, and it would cause a negative financial impact on the business without creating any business value. Interoperability of data analytics tools must be considered when picking a partner and big data technology to avoid creating a giant clutter and to control the foundation that is going to become table stakes of digital instrumentation.

4.1.3.1 Criteria of selection

What criteria should be applied to decide on selecting the appropriate big data and analytics tools to synthesize end-to-end solutions? It necessitates various, disparate tools that have the capability to be integrated together. Multiple tools are required to meet the requirements to deliver a big data analytics platform.

This really depends on several aspects, but it is mainly related to the type of consequences and whether the desired analysis is traditional BI analytics, such as descriptive and predictive analytics, or advanced prescriptive analytics.

The architecture of advanced big data analytics must run in a parallel computing environment with enormous processors to deliver real-time analytics. It should have agility, elasticity, scalability, availability, and security features to accommodate business needs and innovation.

MoSCoW is used to rank the criteria requirements that categorize them into for classes:

M: Must have as the required criteria
S: Should have identified the preferred criteria
C: Could have as an optional criterion if it does not cause impact
W: Won't have now but would like to have it later.

This method of selection allows the prioritization and helps in understanding the needs to choose the adequate tools (Alshehri & Benedicenti, 2013).

The criteria for big data and analytics tools are listed in Table 4.6.

TABLE 4.6 Criteria of selection for big data and analytics

CRITERIA	*MUST HAVE*	*SHOULD HAVE*	*COULD HAVE*	*WON'T HAVE*
Data catalog	X			
ETL/ELT	X			
Data modeling	X			
Meta data management	X			
Data preparation	X			
Data integration	X			
Connectivity to source of data		X		
Data analytics	X			
Advanced analytics	X			
Same platform for data and big data				X
Visualization	X			
Reporting	X			
Automation		X		
Security	X			
Cloud			X	

Other measures should also be taken into consideration when selecting the big data and analytics tools to help implement a successful solution, such as speed and efficiency, ease of use, ease of creation, and ease of integration, which are available in cloud technology.

4.1.3.2 Function of the tools

The function of the tools should be to synthesize a solution that works together collectively into one enterprise platform that is managed and governed to deliver value.

Security and HIPAA privacy rules are deal-breakers in selecting tools that comply with their requirements. The tools should be able to log all activities for auditing purposes. All data communication from the data source must be encrypted, and only authorized users must be allowed to access the data.

Built-in data integration to enable importing comma separated value (CSV) and XML format files, and the ability to perform multithread data loading are essential functions with the flexibility for data preparation to allow renaming, dividing, or creating columns. It is recommended to include data masking features to hide or encrypt confidential data.

A data storage management function that can handle different data types, such as documents, text, log files, images, audio, and video, is required to provide detailed information about the source of data.

The tools need to support the application programming interface (API), which allows applications to interact with each other, and the software development kit (SDK), which includes a set of modules and instructions for developing software. This function delivers a user portal to the enterprise in web services and mobile application formats.

Database function that manages multi-services for SQL and NoSQL for big data and no-ETL analytics in real time. In addition to online analytical processing (OLAP) connectivity, the tools must have a connection to HDFS and text files via third-party product or Apache Hive/Spark.

Moreover, it must be capable of supporting data extraction for relational queries via Open Database Connectivity (ODBC) and Java Database Connectivity (JDBC) drivers. One tool functions as a data pipeline to handle activities in the data factory while generating extract, transform, load (ETL) and extract, load, transform (ELT) jobs and workflows. It is used to clean and ingest data sets to prepare them for processing in a group instead of running them separately.

The analytics tool is a crucial component, and it needs to be compatible with the storage and data lake used in the platform and solution. The outcomes of the analytics tool are presented using a visualization tool, with an easy way to publish in reports or dashboards. Dashboards are utilized to present the results in several interactive chart formats, such as histograms, box plots, heat maps, and tree maps.

HCOs should not waste any of their data. Big data is typically not used by businesses to generate value, but eventually, it can be shared with external consumers for profit. Thus, big data analytics is a business service that requires planning and following data product management methodology to define the roadmap, which involves selecting the technology, providing end-to-end solutions, service support, and a product lifecycle for continuous improvements and adding capabilities.

The framework of the solution design of big data analytics consists of several components considered the building blocks of big data analytics: Infrastructure, platform, data, application software, accessibility, and security.

Networking, compute, and storage are the needed infrastructure for big data analytics. Data is stored in storage and transferred from one host to another via a high-speed network. High-performance computing with a powerful central processing unit (CPU) is an essential driver for big data analytics for real-time results. Databases, big data, and analytics tools are platforms for performing big data analytics. Software applications are part of the foundation of the framework, as they are considered the source of the data generated that we want to analyze. Accessibility in real time to big data analytics from anywhere and from any device is a critical component of the solution design. Security and privacy are built into the design to protect the data and the system's information. All the previous components introduce enormous challenges to the IT department of the HCO.

Emerging technologies such as cloud computing can overcome many of these barriers. It is highly recommended that cloud technology be used to benefit from its agility for fast delivery of business needs and its elasticity to scale up dynamically or down based on business demands. Therefore, cloud technology is suitable for innovative products or services to allow the business to determine if they are viable with managed costs. Thus, enabling big data analytics is a good candidate for cloud computing. Cloud services have various cloud models such as Infrastructure-as-a-Service (IaaS), Platform-as-a-Service (PaaS), and Software-as-a-Service (SaaS). These cloud services could be built on premises as a private cloud, hosted off-site in a colocation, or at a partner data center. The real benefit of cloud technology is obtained when the public cloud is used in a multi-tenant concept that allows several customers to share the same resources in a secure and privacy model without paying for the entire infrastructure cost, as they are billed based on the usage of cloud resources. Public cloud is the most economical way to deploy big data analytics, and it enables IT to use infrastructure in a composable approach as well as big data analytics applications in a modular fashion that is easy to customize and directly consumed with self-service, instead of launching a huge farm of compute powers that can cost a fortune. Additionally, IT can combine private and public clouds into hybrid clouds to exploit both worlds. Thus, the concept of clouds is the same regardless of whether it is private, public, or hybrid.

Consequently, cloud computing plays a vital role in the design of big data analytics solutions, and this initiative should align with the overall comprehensive cloud strategy rather than being an ad hoc initiative led by the analytics team.

4.1.3.2.1 Value proposition

The key value proposition of adopting the framework is to optimize the benefit of big data technology when implemented to allow accessing the patient's "complete" data in real-time to enrich efficiencies in care delivery during the patient's treatment journey. Additionally, it supports the end-to-end pathway and workflow for better patient engagement. It also increases the patient's access to the digital front door experience. Therefore, it is not only cutting the cost of healthcare, but it also adds to the revenue through new business opportunities.

HCOs strive for integrated solutions that focus on driving productivity, efficiency, analytics, and new capabilities such as digital front door and visual care to acquire new patients through new fueling innovation technology-centric offerings like Tele-health, remote patient monitoring, virtual hospital, senior care, and population health that are powered by data technology. Providers and clinicians will be empowered with self-service capabilities in system tools that streamline how they treat patients to be more productive in a mobile fashion.

An essential part of the value proposition is the enabler perspective that is helping to drive quality regulatory to get recognized as a leader organization in healthcare, such as Leapfrog or Watson's top 100 hospitals, which is incredibly powerful for a marketing perspective for growth and strengthening economics. The key benchmarking measures against other HCOs are mortality, readmissions, and acquired infections. Therefore, the value drives quality that cultivates expertise on leveraging new data and advanced analytics to improve the patient journey while being cured. Additionally, it can drive a differentiated patient experience with a flexible scale and an architecturally digital platform around data analytics.

The use of data analytic technologies is to transform the business model toward digital business to provide new revenue and value producing opportunities by evolving traditional HCOs to become a composable Healthcare to be able to compete with retail providers that started to pouring billions of dollars into building digital capabilities as they enter healthcare business while offering a low cost on the continuum of care services. Many retail providers have decided to expand their pharmacy and optometry care to offer other healthcare services such as virtual care retail clinics, health screenings, primary care, and vaccinations with price transparency.

Therefore, for traditional HCO to have market growth and market share gains through new digital products and services, they need to accelerate their digital capabilities and data analytics which, allows the HCO to outreach to primary care physicians (PCPs) to be part of the community connect for mutuel benefit and to encourage other HCO through joint ventures and partnerships acquisitions for larger market share.

Readmissions is another challenge that many HCOs are dealing with when they treat patients outside their network as they cannot ensure that those patients do a follow up with their PCP and they end up getting readmitted again after few days. CMS apply penalties and fines against readmission for not treating outside network patients as their owns patients. A solution such as wearable devices using IoT for tethering remote patient monitoring to stay in touch is a great example of using data analytics throughout the entire patient treatment cycle.

Patient engagement via texting and emails for advice and counsel before patients even come to visit a specialist helps establish a relationship between the doctor, the nurse, and the patient that allows patient education about their illness. Getting data back is incredibly valuable, as it creates a stronger bond with patients, as it almost always communicates with caregivers and their patients. HCOs desire to drive patient experience throughout the treatment journey and improve each touchpoint and interaction for an excellent patient experience throughout their lifetime. Process automation that can save hiring workers to do the same job, but manually.

4.1.4 Cost Analysis

This section aims to identify the total cost of ownership (TCO) of the big data analytics initiative for the lighthouse project without determining the return on investment (ROI), as it is irrelevant in this case. The analysis assesses the gain of achieving the goals that will turn into benefits or business values and determines if it is worth the time and money needed to implement the solution on a larger scale.

Utilizing public cloud is an ongoing operational cost, and HCOs do not need to finance the procurement of hardware infrastructure, such as networking, compute, and storage, using their capital funds. Additionally, most software companies offer subscription-based licenses for their applications and tools in the cloud, which is also considered an operation cost rather than selling perpetual licenses.

The TCO) of a big data analytics product is calculated based on its life cycle and roadmap. A product's life cycle starts with the planning phase and ends when it retires or is replaced.

Walterbusch et al. (2013) provided their respective TCOs of different cloud computing models. The TCO covers the five phases of the product life cycle:

1. The cost of the initiation phase, which involves deciding on the cloud type(s) and services.
2. The cost of the evaluation phase to select the right cloud service provider based on service level agreement (SLA), technology, security, and price requirements.
3. The cost of the transition phase includes implementation and configuration of the services.
4. The cost of the operation phase to run and maintain the service for monitoring and reporting the performance and metered usage charges.

The paper did not include the cost for the dissolution phase as the service can be stopped at any time without penalty. However, if the data stored in the cloud is critical and it needs to be transferred back, then it will be a cost associated with data migration.

As seen in equation 4.1, the TCO of big data analytics is calculated to include the initial cost as capital expenditure (CapEx) and the ongoing cost of operational expenditure (OpEx).

The CapEx includes the consulting and professional fees to implement the project, as many HCOs lack the technical expertise necessary for deployment.

The OpEx includes two variable costs and two fixed costs (equation 4.2). The monthly charges of the connectivity to the cloud (Con_i) and the monthly charges of the cloud services usage (Cld_i) vary each month based on usage with a range from $i = 1$ (first month) to $i = n$ (last month). The two fixed charges are the monthly charges of the software license subscription (Sft), and the monthly labor cost (Lab).

$$\text{TCO} = \text{CapEx} + \text{OpEx} \tag{4.1}$$

where

$$\text{OpEx} = \boldsymbol{Sft} + \boldsymbol{Lab} + \sum_{i=1}^{n} \boldsymbol{Con}_i + \sum_{i=1}^{n} \boldsymbol{Cld}_i \tag{4.2}$$

Even though software vendors and cloud providers offer great help to educate their customers, hiring a consultant to look after the best interests of the HCO is highly recommended. The consultant can provide guidance and direction to select the appropriate technology and cloud services provider. The consulting fee for big data analytics is typically a flat rate of around \$30,000.00, but it can vary based on the length of engagement. Although it can go for several hundred thousand dollars if a distinguished consulting firm is hired to construct a complete digital and cloud strategy. Professional service is needed to implement the solution by subject matter experts (SMEs) in cloud technologies, databases, big data, analytics, data warehousing, and security, with an estimated 120 hours to complete the job at \$250.00 per hour for \$30,000.00. Therefore, the total estimated CapEx is \$60,000.00.

The main portion of the OpEx budget is for the cloud, and it was decided based on an estimated calculator that the public cloud providers supplied online (*Microsoft Website – Azure Pricing Calculator*, n.d.) Table 4.7 shows an itemized list of the components needed for advanced analytics for the lighthouse project, which requires 1 TB of big data and costs \$13,285.50

TABLE 4.7 Estimated cost of big data analytics in public cloud

SERVICE TYPE	*DESCRIPTION*	*ESTIMATED MONTHLY COST*
Azure Synapse Analytics	Tier: Compute optimized Gen2, dedicated SQL pools: DWU 500 × 730 hours, 1 TB of storage with geo-redundant disaster recovery	$5,592.05
Azure Data Factory	Azure data factory V2 type, data pipeline service type, Azure integration runtime: 100 activity runs, 100 data movement units, 10,000 pipeline activities, 10,000 pipeline activities—external, self-hosted integration runtime: 100 activity runs, 1,000 data movement units, 10,000 pipeline activities, 10,000 pipeline activities—External, data flow: 1 × 8 compute optimized vCores × 730 hours, 1 × 8 general purpose vCores × 730 hours, 1 × 8 memory optimized vCores × 730 hours, data factory operations: 100 × 50,000 read/write operations, 100 × 50,000 monitoring operations	$5,045.12
Azure Analysis Services	Developer (hours), 1 instance(s), 720 hours	$95.04
Power BI Embedded	1 node(s) × 720 hours, node type: A2, 2 virtual core(s), 5 GB RAM, 301–600 peak renders/hour	$1,445.83
Storage Accounts	Block blob storage, general purpose V2, LRS redundancy, hot access tier, 1,000 GB capacity—pay as you go, 100,000 write operations, 100,000 list and create container operations, 100,000 read operations, 100,000 archive high priority read, 1 other operations. 1,000 GB data retrieval, 1,000 GB archive high priority retrieval, 1,000 GB data write	$19.44
Azure Databricks	All-purpose compute workload, premium tier, 1 D3V2 (4 vCPU(s), 14 GB RAM) × 730 hours, pay as you go, 0.75 DBU × 730 hours	$504.80
Azure Cosmos DB	Standard provisioned throughput (manual), single region write (Single-Master)—East US (Write Region); 400 RU/s × 730 hours; 1,000 GB transactional storage, 2 copies of periodic backup storage; Dedicated gateway not enabled	$273.36

(*Continued*)

TABLE 4.7 Estimated cost of big data analytics in public cloud (*Continued*)

SERVICE TYPE	*DESCRIPTION*	*ESTIMATED MONTHLY COST*
Virtual Machines	1 D2 v3 (2 vCPUs, 8 GB RAM) × 730 hours; Windows—(OS only); Pay as you go; 0 managed disks—S4, 100 transaction units; inter region transfer type, 5 GB outbound data transfer from West US to East Asia	$152.62
Virtual Network	1,000 GB data transfer from East US region to East US region	$20.00
Cloud Services	1 D2 v3 (2 Core(s), 8 GB RAM) × 730 hours	$137.24
	Total	**$13,285.50**

monthly. Human labor is also part of OpEx, and about 50 hours a month at $50 per hour are expected for operation support, for a total of $2500. Thus, the total monthly OpEx is about $15,785.50.

4.1.5 Expected Outcomes

The expected outcomes of the framework allow the use of appropriate technology to provide high accuracy of a complete medical record (volume and depth) and enhance clinical documentation necessary to attain system-wide quality in real time and revenue targets.

The revenue depends on accurate documentation that ensures appropriate reimbursement and collections against denials. As the healthcare reimbursement model is changing, causing fines for HCOs with lower quality of care, embracing the framework shall prevent inadequate patient treatment by alerting providers to the severity of illness with complete health records to prevent making wrong conclusions that reduce the risk of mortality of the patients. Moreover, CMS decides the reimbursement rates to hospitals for Medicare and Medicaid patients by applying the Case Mix Index (CMI), which is a metric that evokes the mixture, difficulty, and seriousness of diseases of patients treated at an HCO facility.

Additionally, it will eliminate the manual process of reviewing the clinical documentation, as many HCOs have a challenge of reviewing 100% of charts, which may cause a missed opportunity for prospective payment to maximize reimbursement by classifying patients with an inappropriate

Diagnosis-Related Group (DRG). This allows automation to review charts to support case management throughout the patient's stay until discharge, with the length of stay (LOS) information.

The expected outcomes when having big data as part of data completeness for analytics. In addition to reimbursement and quality, it adds automation and real-time reporting capabilities as expected outcomes.

1. **Reimbursement**: ensure clinical documentation conditions have adequate backing proof to maximize CMI
2. **Quality**: benchmarks for recognizing the difficulty of treating patient illness within HCOs.
3. **Automation**: process and workflow for Parallel and retrospective evaluations
4. **Real-time reporting**: real-time DRG and patient LOS information

4.1.6 Implementation of Framework

The benefit of adopting a framework for HCOs is to avoid rolling out a tool or a system that does not meet the needs to accomplish the expected outcomes. If a well-defined methodology is fundamentally used correctly, it will lead to successful results. Many HCOs do not recognize the process aspect or the skill and competence aspects of their technical team and focus only on the tools. HCOs can spend money on software applications and designate the time and resources. Still, it cannot create a ROI if they are not focused on putting all parts of the puzzle together to work coherently.

The objective of the case study is to support implementing the framework to employ big data to add capabilities such as automation, image deep learning, ML, and AI to HCOs. The need is to enhance the use of the available data and analytic tools and try to eliminate what is not working or fitting.

The framework took multiple years to be implemented in one of the HCOs in the state of Florida with the following profile:

- $4.3B annual revenue
- 3,200-bed system
- 15 hospitals and emergency departments
- 4,200 physicians
- 80 medical specialties and subspecialties
- 22,000 team members
- 150,000 inpatients and nearly 3.1 million outpatients.

The implementation of the framework started in 2018 by identifying the necessary elements to revamp the entire data strategy that addresses the challenges of the HCO. It required a full IT transformation and organization restructuring that permits partnering with the business, rather than being a technology service provider, to ensure alignment with this HCO's six strategic imperatives:

1. Embrace quality and safety
2. Become best place to work
3. Earn physician loyalty
4. Drive growth and innovation
5. Enhance ease of use
6. Strengthen economics.

Like other HCOs in the healthcare industry, this HCO realized the change of healthcare regulatory from pay-for-service to pay-for-value aiming to deliver high-quality healthcare at a lower cost with great experience for both patients and providers. The solution of those challenges is to leverage the fully available data, including semi-structured and unstructured data, for better analytics in the clinical and business areas to make data driven decisions in real-time utilizing emerging technologies.

As background, the initial evaluation revealed the inconsistency of the applications with exacerbated silos because of the lack of standardization. Despite the number of analytic tools and their high TCO, it was obvious that the organization's data capabilities had been suffering because of the gap in the technical skills of the available tools for data analytics. Both data and analytics functions were controlled by IT, which led to other departments and business units establishing what is called "shadow IT". As a result of a lack of coordination, too many data analytics tools and systems of the same function were found, which added to the operational expenses with no tangible benefits.

Additionally, this model caused delays in making decisions in clinical and business matters due to spending more time piecing several outputs together.

Furthermore, the design of the data analytic system and its follow-up were very complicated and least desirable, leading to a low-performance and unstable system.

Regarding data sources, the finding showed that the HCO used 1,275+ applications that generated 3,339 TB of data, of which 436 applications were identified as the core of the ecosystem that the HCO used as a source of data for reporting and data analytics for clinical and non-clinical areas, as shown in Table 4.8.

TABLE 4.8 List of system applications

AREA	*CLINICAL SYSTEM*	*NUMBER OF APPLICATIONS*
Clinical	Allied health	92
	In/Outpatient	30
	Inpatient	78
	Outpatient	49
	Population health	4
	Clinical Total	**253**
Non-Clinical	HIM	28
	Patient access	24
	Patient experience	3
	ERP	27
	Others	101
	Non-Clinical Total	**183**
	Total	**436**

Additionally, this HCO is participating in One-Florida and HIE for exchanging data and health information with CMS and other HCOs in the region

4.1.6.1 Analytics tools

Eighty-four embedded and stand-alone analytics applications and tools were identified with more than 11,000 data elements that provide reporting and BI across 38 business units. The annual cost of licensing and supporting these analytics applications is $5,783,630.00. The list of analytics applications includes QlikView, Tableau, Power BI, IBM SPSS, Crystal Reports, SQL Server Reporting Service (SSRS), and a third-party vendor of EDW. In addition, about 20+ other analytics applications were identified as analytics applications but were not included in the analytics application's portfolio. However, many applications hosted on-premises with outdated technology presented security and support risks to the enterprise without delivering the best value to the business. Furthermore, the cost of these applications is very high, and the ROI is very low due to the fragmented and poor overall performance of the analytics application's portfolio.

Moreover, users needed extensive training to use the applications, which kept them away from their core business of healthcare.

TABLE 4.9 List of analytics tools

BUSINESS UNIT AREA	*NUMBER OF APPLICATIONS*
Administration	2
Audit Compliance	4
Care Assessment and Discharge	1
Care Delivery	40
Care Initiation/Registration	1
Care Management	6
Billing and Reporting	1
Encounter Initiation/Scheduling	1
Finance	20
Human Resources	1
Legal	1
Medical Education and Research	3
Performance Management	1
Regulatory	2
Revenue Cycle	8
Supply Chain	2

Table 4.9 indicates the analytic tools for reporting and BI using the data sourced from the HCO's ecosystem applications.

In 2018, Health Catalyst Enterprise Data Warehouse (EDW) had approximately 8.8 TB of data from 14 source systems for analytics with 50% compression ratio, includes both the database and indexes. Total environment footprint includes OS and data on all servers including the EDW and audit servers which consume most of the data. Health Catalyst's EDW is not a system of record or archive platform for source systems, databases or applications and the HCO is keeping its existing data sources separate from the EDW if additional data elements need to be extracted to EDW. QlikView hybrid licensees' model is used for visualizations with inadequate data flow and limited accessibility for users at the HCO side.

The primary challenge of the HCO is how to stop spending money on data and analytic tools that are silos, redundant, and almost outdated.

Implementing the framework has allowed the HCO to overcome this issue and it has offered the principles of revamping the entire data strategy with a new fragmented landscape for data investment. It started with people aspect as IT was formed in a function and/or a role structure to support the use of technology at the HCO. The applications team acted as a function maintaining the data warehouse and dealt with data integration tasks in a responsive manner to the clinical and business areas that request reports and KPIs information.

The role of the applications team members depended on their skillsets to execute the set of assignments and their availability to deliver the reports needed. Thus, the IT structure for data related areas limits the HCO from being proactive to achieve the data strategy.

Applying the framework allowed addressing the challenges with data being disparate and moving away from the center focus of the organization because of the high cost and complexity.

At the People layer, the change of the organization structure presented an explicit focus on data as a product that drives toward an enterprise level, rather than having business unites apply Do-It-Yourself (DIY) approach when it comes to leveraging data analytics and creating reports.

It started with appointing a CDAIO who has a healthcare acumen with a big picture mentality and strategic agility to allow collaboration between business units and IT. The role of the CDAIO is to oversee the venture capital in the data and analytics technologies to align opportunities and investments. Additionally, leading the data team that is responsible for business analysis, enterprise analytics and data science with defined job descriptions. In addition to the CDAIO, four leadership positions were needed to support the direction of the HCO's data strategy as functional areas.

A data product manager is a new role that shepherds possible opportunity using data from the starting idea to execution and it was created to develop guidelines for managing the data products for enhancement and operational support to reach a level of product maturity with standardization and product life cycle for new releases. In addition, establishing product roadmap and setting KPIs are key tasks for the data product owner that involved showing the success of the data product and value realization.

At the organization level, the CDAIO worked with the HCO's executive leadership to align data strategy with the quality and performance of the organization overall strategy by innovation. That required collaboration with other business unites for a new fragmented data and analytics landscape that serves patients and drives for growing market shares.

At the process layer, an effort was made to revamp the processes around data owners, data stewards, and data custodians for data governance attainment that aligns with business processes. The goal is to enable the organization with data transparency where accuracy and trust data are easy to access and data literacy where users can read, communicate, and understand the data, resulting in value. Data governance is essential to ensure transparent choices and responsibilities regarding data decisions. It classifies the needed decisions, who makes them, and how they are made.

1. Data privacy involves controlling access and encrypting the data to ensure that it is secured and only accessed by the right users.
2. Data management involves keeping the data arranged and structured for usability according to policy and procedure.
3. Data lifecycle classifies the data into active, archive, delete, and purge.
4. Data quality means being confident in the data available and that it suits the purpose of usage.
5. Data ownership is to identify the department that is accountable for the data assets that the department generates.
6. Data valuation is to deliver full value data analytics that align with the strategy.

At the technology layer, by focusing on a subgroup of legacy analytics tools that have outdated technology and need to be checked to remediate risk and lower costs, the framework aided in optimizing the analytics applications portfolio by standardization, which allowed eliminating 9% of duplicate analytics tools and saving about $1.4 M in licenses and support.

Furthermore, modernized applications were added to the data and analytics applications portfolio to migrate toward an enterprise platform that takes advantage of the contemporary software offered in the cloud, supporting predictive analytics and utilizing the available structured and unstructured data.

Figure 4.5 shows the layout of the migrated data and analytics platform shifting toward cloud computing.

The solution is designed to be modeled as building blocks in a composable fashion that can be assembled or reassembled, and the ability to expand based on selected functions and tool abilities to meet business goals.

The applications that supply data are location-independent and distributed in several places: on-premises, vendor-hosted, and public cloud. Additionally, Health Catalyst has remained a vendor of the EDW hosted in its tenant in Azure cloud, which offers innovative data warehousing platforms.

The analytics functions are performed in the cloud as a SaaS, and they only require checking a box or clicking on the desired functionality.

This solution effectively placed data completeness into the hands of the business with insignificant interaction from users when executing data analytics jobs.

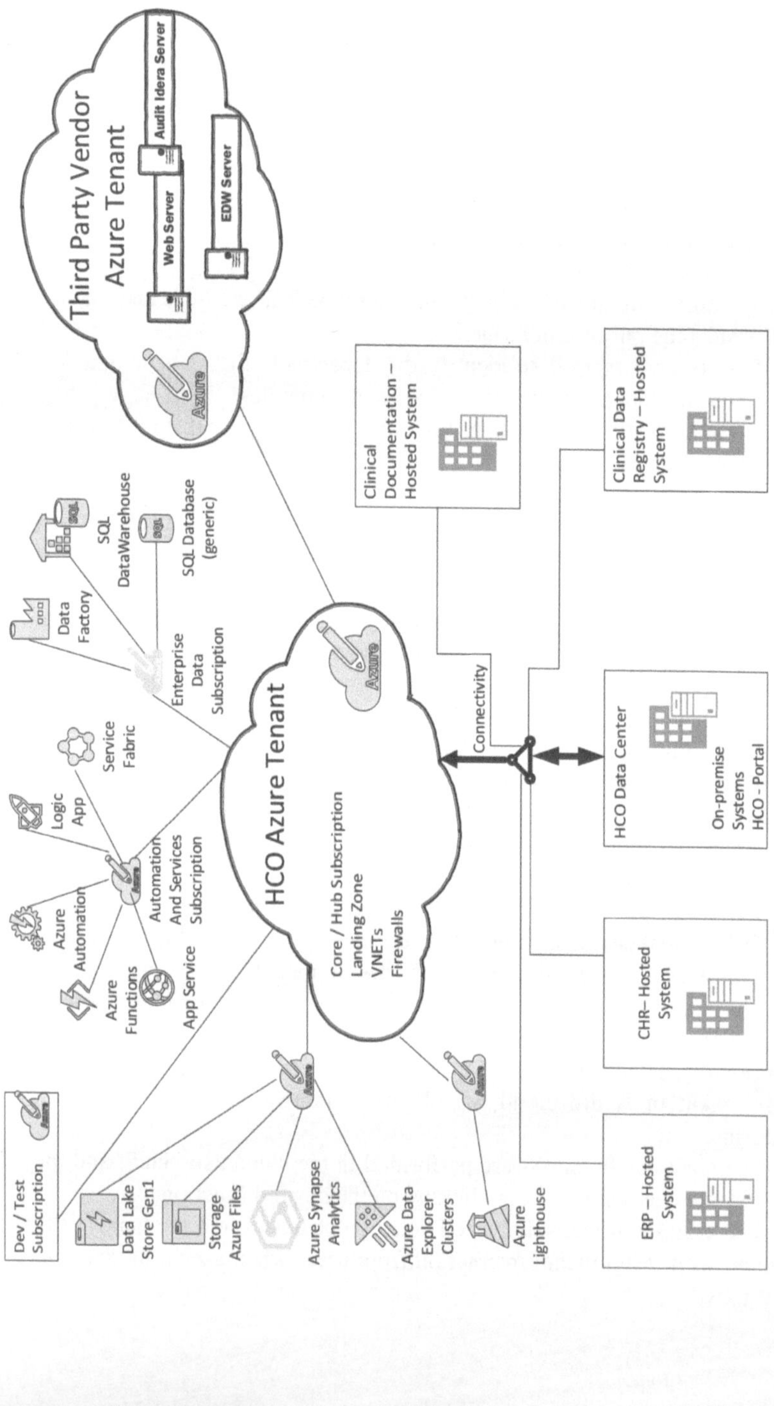

FIGURE 4.5 Modernized data and analytics platform transformation—A composable architecture.

REFERENCES

Adjerid, I., Adler-Milstein, J., & Angst, C. J. (2018). Reducing medicare spending through electronic health information exchange: The role of incentives and exchange maturity. *Information Systems Research*, *29*(2), 341–361.

Almotairi, M. (2009). A framework for successful CRM implementation. *European and Mediterranean Conference on Information Systems (pp. 1–12).*

Alshehri, S., & Benedicenti, L. (2013). Using the analytical hierarchy process as a ranking tool for user story prioritization techniques. *Proceedings of the 8th International Conference on Software Engineering Advances.*

Brugha, R., & Varvasovszky, Z. (2000). Stakeholder analysis: A review. *Health Policy and Planning*, *15*(3), 239–246.

Cates, J. E., Gill, S. S., & Zeituny, N. (2005). The ladder of business intelligence (LOBI): A framework for enterprise IT planning and architecture. *International Journal of Business Information Systems*, *1*(1–2), 220–238.

ECRI Website. (n.d.). https://www.ecri.org/

HealthIT.gov Website. (n.d.). https://www.healthit.gov/topic/health-it-and-health-information-exchange-basics/what-hie

Hu, J., & Nerenz, D. R. (2020). Performance of multihospital health systems' flagship hospitals in the CMS Star Rating Program. *Journal of Hospital Medicine*, *15*(7), 407–410.

Klotz, L., Horman, M., Bi, H. H., & Bechtel, J. (2008). The impact of process mapping on transparency. *International Journal of Project Management*, 57(8), 623–636.

McCurdy, R. K. (2001). A Comparison of the Audit and Accreditation Tools Used by the Health Care Financing Administration, The Texas Department of Insurance, and The National Committee on Quality Assurance: The Cost of Multi-Agency Oversight on Medicare + Choice Plans in Texas.

Microsoft Website – Azure Pricing calculator. (n.d.). https://azure.microsoft.com/en-us/pricing/calculator/

Nelson, E. C., Homa, K., Mastanduno, M. P., Fisher, E. S., Batalden, P. B., & Malcolm, E. F. (2005). Publicly reporting comprehensive quality and cost data: A health care system's transparency initiative. *Patient Safety*, *31*(10), 573–584.

Ouayogodé, M. H., Colla, C. H., & Lewis, V. A. (2017). Determinants of success in shared savings programs: An analysis of ACO and market characteristics. *Healthcare*, *5*(1–2), 53–61. Elsevier.

Parkash, S., & Kaushik, V. K. (2011). Supplier performance monitoring and improvement (SPMI) through SIPOC analysis and PDCA model to the ISO 9001 QMS in sports goods manufacturing industry. *Journal of Leadership, LogForum* *7*(4).

Sarkar, A., Mukhopadhyay, A. R., & Ghosh, S. K. (2011). Selection of Critical Processes for "process improvement." *International Journal of Lean Six Sigma*, 2(4), 356–370.

Sony, M., Antony, J., & Douglas, J. A. (2020). Essential ingredients for the implementation of quality 4.0: A narrative review of literature and future directions for research. *The TQM Journal*, 32(4), 779–793.

Sullivan, T. (2017). Epic's rival EHR vendors say they too are making the "CHR" switch. *Healthcare IT News*.

Tortorella, G. L., Fogliatto, F. S., Mac Cawley Vergara, A., Vassolo, R., & Sawhney, R. (2020). Healthcare 4.0: Trends, challenges and research directions. *Production Planning and Control*, *31*(15). https://doi.org/10.1080/09537287.2019.1702226

Trebble, T. M., Hansi, N., Hydes, T., Smith, M. A., & Baker, M. (2010). Process mapping the patient journey: An introduction. *BMJ*, *341*.

Walterbusch, M., Martens, B., & Teuteberg, F. (2013). Evaluating cloud computing services from a total cost of ownership perspective. *Management Research Review*, 36(6), 613–638.

Healthcare Big Data Framework 5

Architecture, Deployment, and SME Validation

A framework is a structured representation of interconnected and cohesive processes designed to accomplish a complex task. It defines *what* must be done to develop a solution that effectively coordinates the efforts of all essential components, ensuring value creation and alignment with business objectives. However, before adoption, it is critical to rigorously evaluate and validate the framework to confirm that it justifies the investment of time and resources.

5.1 SYSTEM ARCHITECTURE OF THE FRAMEWORK

The system architecture provides a structured blueprint describing the physical layout and relationships among complex system components. This architectural view is essential in healthcare big data analytics to ensure consistency,

DOI: 10.1201/9781003610731-5

standardization, and alignment with organizational goals. Steiner (1998) emphasizes that effective architecture goes beyond technical specifications to convey how system components interact within a holistic framework.

Architecting a healthcare system involves integrating multi-disciplinary components into a cohesive model that supports full system development. This method requires consideration of multiple domains and views to guide decisions during implementation. According to Maier (1996), the representation of a system through various "views" facilitates understanding its structure and behavior. These six views—Purpose/Objectives, Behavior, Managerial, Form, Performance, and Data—enable stakeholders to explore different dimensions of the system, from strategic intent to operational capability.

Organizing architectural components and connectors into coherent styles enhances system functionality while clearly defining boundaries and constraints. Each architectural style—characterized by specific interaction patterns among its elements—embodies distinct capabilities and limitations that shape the system's overall behavior and performance.

The proposed system architecture for healthcare organizations (HCOs) integrates five interconnected domains: business, process, technology, application, and data architectures. This holistic model aligns with enterprise goals for deploying big data solutions.

1. **Business Architecture** sets a strategic direction, encompassing vision, service capabilities, operating models, and performance metrics. It embeds regulatory compliance and outlines stakeholder roles and structures, fostering a culture of innovation and accountability.
2. **Process Architecture** defines the workflows and activities governing the data lifecycle, including access, sharing, and privacy protection. It establishes dynamic governance protocols that ensure security and efficiency.
3. **Technology Architecture** comprises hardware infrastructure, network protocols, and cloud environments. It delineates the standards for computing, storage, and edge devices, such as biomedical sensors and IoT systems, all integrated with cybersecurity safeguards.
4. **Application Architecture** includes the applications, databases, and user interfaces that support healthcare analytics. It must deliver intuitive user experiences while maintaining compatibility across platforms.
5. **Data Architecture** serves as the cornerstone, linking all other layers. It governs data integration, ingestion, cleansing, validation, curation,

cataloging, and lineage tracking. The enterprise data hub unifies structured (data warehouse) and unstructured (data lake) information, while virtualization provides seamless, real-time data delivery.

Advanced analytics—such as machine learning (ML), natural language processing (NLP), and data mining—derive insights from curated data. These insights are translated into action through various processing modes (transaction, batch, or stream). Results are presented through interactive visualizations, dashboards, and traditional business intelligence tools, empowering stakeholders with real-time, data-driven decision-making.

This architectural model serves as a technical roadmap and a strategic asset, ensuring resilience, adaptability, and performance across HCOs.

Figure 5.1 shows the big data analytics system architecture comprising the five sub-architectures with their components. At the strategic level, the Business architecture ensures alignment with regulatory standards, strategic goals, and stakeholder needs. At the same time, the Process Architecture governs the data lifecycle, management, and security, which is critical for healthcare compliance and quality. The Technology Architecture supports scalability and interoperability through diverse endpoints (e.g., IoT, biomedical devices) and cloud-based infrastructure with embedded security mechanisms. The Application Architecture facilitates data interaction through clinical, analytical, and business tools, backed by relational and non-relational databases designed for optimized user experiences. These layers converge in the System Architecture, which orchestrates a powerful big data Architecture pipeline encompassing data ingestion, cleansing, storage, and analysis using ML, NLP, and real-time processing. Outputs are delivered via dashboards and reports that drive actionable clinical insights, predictions, and informed decision-making. The architecture's layered and modular design ensures scalability, adaptability, and value creation, making it a vital framework for modern, data-driven healthcare systems.

5.2 DEPLOYMENT

To test and validate the proposed framework, we selected an existing, well-established HCO that operates multiple hospitals and employs over 10,000 staff members. Throughout the study, this organization will be referred to as HCO. HCO served as the site for implementing a lighthouse project—a proof of concept (PoC) designed to assess the feasibility and value of new technologies within a digital transformation context. This strategic approach enabled the

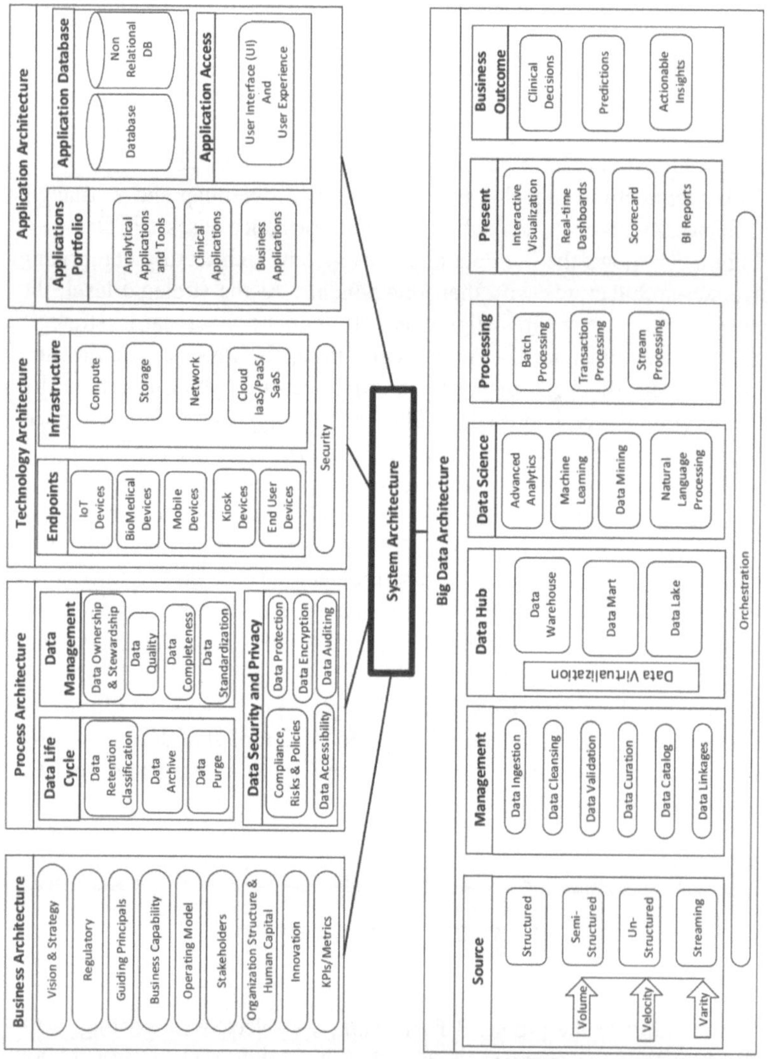

FIGURE 5.1 Layered system architecture for healthcare, integrating business, process, technology, and application domains.

evaluation of key performance metrics, helping determine whether the initiative warranted further scaling or should be discontinued early, thereby reducing the risk of wasted investment. While immediate improvements were not guaranteed, the lighthouse project provided a baseline success threshold, opening pathways for innovation, operational efficiency, and data-informed decision-making.

To ensure the initiative's success, HCO launched the lighthouse project with a fusion team, following the model recommended by Gartner (2019). This cross-functional team brought together professionals from administration, business units, clinical informatics, IT, vendors, and business analytics, all under the guidance of a delivery manager. The team focused on delivering integrated value across the organization, avoiding the pitfalls of siloed efforts and redundant analytics initiatives. The fusion team also played a critical role in aligning the project with HCO's broader enterprise architecture, setting strategic goals and managing resources and governance structures to enable sustainable, scalable, and coherent innovation across different business areas.

5.3 EXERCISE THE SYSTEM

In healthcare, value is represented with several qualitative and quantitative measures for financial and non-financial metrics, including tangible and intangible. The tangible assets such as buildings, equipment, and inventories are 15% of the organization's value in today's economy.

The intangible assets are not translated to monetary value but are essential to show the framework's benefits. Some intangible measurements are accreditation, reputation, awards/recognitions, patient engagement/loyalty/satisfaction, and physicians' satisfaction. Value in healthcare is classified as access, perceptions, capability, impact, and financial gain, and it should be balanced, efficient, and reliable for tactical and strategic results. Every patient's care journey must be measured, documented, and reported in the healthcare industry, including costs, outputs, quality, time, patient satisfaction, innovation, and HCO reputation.

Volume and market share growth are key values needed for measuring the success of the HCO (Phillips et al., 2013).

With the data analytics complete, the HCO has a better-quality outcome and can create and submit quality reports to the organizations in Table 5.1 more efficiently and promptly.

The improvement in quality care permitted HCO to win the Watson Health 100 Top Hospitals award in 2021. To earn this award, the HCO should have a high-quality survival, a low number of infections, low 30-day readmission, and

TABLE 5.1 Organization for healthcare ranking and awards

QUALITY PROGRAM	*REPORT FREQUENCY*	*BENCHMARKING*	*RISK*	*FINANCIAL METRICS*
CMS Value-Based Purchasing (VBP)	Annually	✓	✓	✓
CMS Reporting Inpatient/ Outpatient	Quarterly	✓	✓	✓
CMS Readmission Reduction	Annually	✓	✓	
CMS Hospital-Acquired Condition (HAC) Reduction Program	Annually	✓	✓	
AHCA (Florida Only)	Biannually	✓ (FL only)		
Watson Health 100	Annually	✓	✓	✓
Leapfrog	Quarterly	✓		
US News & World Report	Annually			
Becker's	Annually			
Healthgrades	Annually	✓		
Comparion	Annually	✓	✓	✓

low 30-day mortality rates. Additional criteria, such as a short wait time in the emergency room, good financial performance, and great patient satisfaction, are also considered in the evaluation. Additionally, an Everest award was granted for the top performance and high rate of improvement over 5 years.

Between 2017 and 2018, this HCO had a 34% market share compared to its competitor in the area, with 45% based on the number provided by the Agency for Health Care Administration (AHCA). Notably, admissions increased from approximately 100,570 in 2016 to over 118,000 in 2019, while patient days and average daily census also showed sustained growth, reflecting improved capacity utilization. Emergency department (ED) patient volume rose steadily, indicating growing demand for acute care services. Although outpatient visits peaked in 2018, the overall volume remained high in 2019, demonstrating HCO's strong engagement across inpatient and outpatient services. These trends highlight the organization's expanding operational footprint and growing ability to efficiently serve a larger patient population. The upward movement across these metrics supports the effectiveness of HCO's strategic investments in infrastructure, digital transformation, and care delivery optimization.

Analytics tools assessment is part of the exercise to evaluate the capability of the tools and their cost. As seen in Table 5.2, the assessment revealed

TABLE 5.2 Cost of analytics tools

ROW LABELS	*SUM OF CALC_TIME_COST_TOTAL*
Eliminated	$8,251,980.92
Business	$6,001,980.92
Reporting/Visualization	$6,001,980.92
Clinical	$1,325,000.00
Reporting/Visualization	$1,325,000.00
ERP	$650,000.00
Reporting/Visualization	$650,000.00
Other	$75,000.00
Reporting/Visualization	$75,000.00
(blank)	$200,000.00
Reporting/Visualization	$200,000.00
No Action	$15,391,503.00
Business	$1,878,750.00
Reporting/Visualization	$1,878,750.00
Clinical	$1,304,375.00
Reporting/Visualization	$1,304,375.00
ERP	$1,373,000.00
Reporting/Visualization	$1,373,000.00
Other	$475,000.00
Reporting/Visualization	$475,000.00
Productivity	$1,683,500.00
Reporting/Visualization	$1,683,500.00
Utility	$725,000.00
Data Science	$575,000.00
Reporting/Visualization	$150,000.00
(blank)	$7,951,878.00
Data Science	$0.00
Don't Know	$350,000.00
Reporting/Visualization	$7,526,878.00
(blank)	$75,000.00

(Continued)

TABLE 5.2 Cost of analytics tools (*Continued*)

ROW LABELS	*SUM OF CALC_TIME_COST_TOTAL*
Retained	$9,199,462.52
Business	$3,100,000.00
Data Science	$50,000.00
Reporting/Visualization	$3,050,000.00
Clinical	$1,650,000.00
Reporting/Visualization	$1,650,000.00
ERP	$2,342,462.52
Data Science	$1,967,462.52
Reporting/Visualization	$375,000.00
Productivity	$25,000.00
Reporting/Visualization	$25,000.00
Utility	$7,000.00
Reporting/Visualization	$7,000.00
(blank)	$2,075,000.00
Reporting/Visualization	$2,075,000.00
Grand Total	$32,842,946.44

that the HCO spends around $33M on analytics tools, and about $8.3M, or about 25% of the total cost, can be reduced by eliminating some of the analytics tools. The HCO spends about $9M on analytics tools with the right technical requirements and fit innovation and advanced analytics. These tools should be retained. Less than half of the spending of $15M needs to be re-engineered and migrated for better use.

In addition to earning prestigious awards and reducing costs by retiring outdated analytics tools, HCO achieved significant financial gains, including a $112 million net income increase in 2018—a 52% rise over 2017—and a 48% increase in net income to $313 million in early 2021 compared to 2019. Revenue grew from $946.79 million in 2019 to $1.08 billion in 2021. These improvements were driven in part by the use of advanced data analytics in emergency departments, which led to a 49% reduction in patients who left without being seen (LWBS), a 92% reduction in patients leaving against medical advice (AMA), faster discharge identification for 20% of cases, and an average discharge time reduction of 17.5 minutes—boosting both operational efficiency and patient satisfaction.

5.4 VALIDATIONS

The validations of the proposed framework in Chapter 4 consist of two methods: a case study and subject matter expert (SME) interviews. The case study examines the framework in a large HCO in Florida, United States.

SMEs also reviewed the big data and analytics framework in healthcare and technology for further validation. Additionally, the qualitative approach forms a profound understanding of the framework while validating it rather than a quantitative method that deals with numbers. Qualitative validation deepens the framework's outcomes by including a multi-dimensional view and answering questions such as how, who, why, where, and when. These provide accurate assessments to demonstrate good results (Leung, 2015).

5.5 CASE STUDY

A case study is a research method that can be used to validate the conceptual framework. The questions of "how" and "why" are possibly being asked to direct the use of case studies to fulfill the principles of the qualitative method to define, comprehend, and explain a real-life execution of a framework (Yin, 2009).

The proposed framework was executed as a real-life case study covered in Chapter 4's Implementation of Framework section. The validation of the case study is examined, and the result of adopting the framework is successful with the expected outcomes.

5.6 INTERVIEWS

A qualitative method was applied to evaluate the proposed framework, using semi-structured interviews with SMEs. This approach enables a deep understanding of complex topics through open-ended questions, and its validity relies on credibility, authenticity, criticality, and integrity (Lincoln & Guba, 1985; Whittemore et al., 2001). Secondary criteria such as vividness, creativity, and congruence, as well as techniques like design consideration and data analysis, further supported methodological rigor. SMEs were selected based on their education and extensive healthcare analytics experience (Pace & Sheehan, 2002). Interviews were designed according to best practices to minimize bias (Teter, 2014), and the number of participants was determined by data saturation, consistent with guidelines by Dworkin (2012) and Yusoff (2019).

5.6.1 Interview Questions

- *Overall, how well do you think the framework overcomes the challenges in big data analytics adoption in healthcare? Follow-up: And why?*
- *What does the framework provide for healthcare organizations that they are NOT currently considering when implementing big data analytics?*
- *What step or function needs to be included in the framework to address any gap?*
- *In your opinion, what will be the most beneficial matter to healthcare organizations when the proposed framework's structured approach is followed?*

A total of 16 SMEs were contacted, with 12 agreeing to participate and 9 completing interviews, reaching saturation. Each interview lasted approximately 30 minutes, was conducted via Microsoft Teams, Zoom, or in person, and was recorded with consent. Transcriptions were cleaned for clarity and anonymity. The average SME had 18.9 years of experience, totaling 170 years across participants. Questions were piloted with two SMEs and reviewed by the faculty of a Major University with expertise in Qualitative Methods, leading to a shift from a structured to a semi-structured format.

5.6.2 Analysis

As seen in Table 5.3, the responses from the nine SMEs were analyzed using thematic analysis (TA) to evaluate the strengths and gaps in the proposed big data analytics framework for healthcare. TA helped identify key patterns and themes, confirming that while the framework effectively addresses major challenges in healthcare data adoption, it must go beyond just technology. SMEs emphasized the importance of including all six framework layers—especially those related to organization, people, and processes—to achieve successful outcomes. Treating data as a product and assigning a product owner was also crucial to value delivery.

TABLE 5.3 Thematic analysis of interviews with subject matter experts (SMEs)

SME	*BACKGROUND*	*FRAMEWORK EFFECTIVENESS (Q1)*	*MISSING IN HCOS (Q2)*	*GAPS IN FRAMEWORK (Q3)*	*BENEFITS (Q4)*
SME #1	BS Computer Science, 16 years. Data Engineer with expertise in business analytics and intelligence.	Yes, it addresses both technical and organizational challenges effectively.	Absence of tech selection committees and lack of implementation detail.	It needs stronger stakeholder engagement and system-level integration.	Promotes enterprise data view, strategic alignment, and focus on business outcomes.
SME #2	BS EE, MS IE, 17 years. Principal Enterprise Architect with a focus on data integration and analytics.	Yes, it aligns well with business pillars and addresses core pain points.	Disconnect between tech and business; people and process misalignment.	Lacks a detailed operational model and forward-looking roadmap.	Clarifies value outcomes, supports IoT integration, and drives innovation.
SME #3	PhD in Healthcare Management, 13 years. R&D Scientist focused on clinical data quality and outcomes.	Yes, it clearly outlines actionable components and stakeholder roles.	Undefined roles for data ownership; lack of metric-driven goals.	It needs implementation and a continuous improvement plan (PDCA).	Breaks silos, improve efficiency, adapts dynamically, and benefits both HCOs and patients.
SME #4	MS in Healthcare Admin, 10 years. Consultant in value-based care, reporting, and forecasting.	Yes, it integrates organizational goals with analytics and reconnects IT and business.	Disconnected data lifecycle, outdated records, missing real-time insights.	Need for training, tool understanding, and standardized definitions.	Forecasting capability, enhanced collaboration, improved operational ROI.
SME #5	PharmD, 24 years. Senior Director in performance, quality, and clinical decision support.	Yes, it highlights data complexity and builds confidence in data governance.	Incomplete data governance limited maturity in data management.	Leadership education on data usage and tool capability gaps.	It improves clinical workflows, enables lifecycle governance, and enhances team effectiveness.

(*Continued*)

TABLE 5.3 Thematic analysis of interviews with subject matter experts (SMEs) (*Continued*)

SME	*BACKGROUND*	*FRAMEWORK EFFECTIVENESS (Q1)*	*MISSING IN HCOS (Q2)*	*GAPS IN FRAMEWORK (Q3)*	*BENEFITS (Q4)*
SME #6	BS CS, MS IT Management, MBA, 20 years. Technical Lead in EMR and enterprise architecture.	It covers core aspects, including data integrity, security, and privacy.	Neglect of data accuracy and comprehensive integration practices.	Lacks innovative elements and a multi-layered perspective.	Empowers patients through data apps and promotes healthy lifestyles via insights.
SME #7	MS MIS, 26 years. Senior Analyst specializing in EMR systems and data analytics.	Yes, it addresses major challenges, including unstructured data and dependencies.	Incomplete data lifecycle processes, weak ownership/ stewardship roles.	Missing NLP integration and defined operational model.	Enables cost reduction, IoT leverage, and better patient experience.
SME #8	24 years. Enterprise Account Manager. Expert in data, AI/ML pipelines for healthcare.	Yes, comprehensive and culturally shift-inducing.	Limited recognition of IoT and data value.	Lacks MVP, audit mechanisms, and rapid feedback loops.	Supports data-driven culture, maps value flow, and enables complete transformation.
SME #9	AS in Computer Science, 20 years. Solutions Architect in modern healthcare data platforms.	Strong foundational support across diverse clinical systems.	Misalignment among clinicians, IT, and business stakeholders.	Missing lineage tracking, data reuse logic, and streaming data features.	Enables predictive, personalized healthcare and improved infrastructure scalability.

However, gaps were identified, particularly in formal training, innovation, PDCA (Plan-Do-Check-Act) practices, and the operational model. Training should be a distinct component within the process layer to ensure competency and real-time decision-making. Innovation, absent from the current framework, should be integrated across organizational, process, and technology domains. PDCA can be embedded within innovation activities as a foundation of continuous improvement. Lastly, SMEs recommended developing an operational model, such as a Concept of Operations (CONOPS), under the responsibility of the data product owner—a potential area for future research.

SMEs emphasized that big data analytics in healthcare is uniquely complex and massive compared to other industries, requiring specialized oversight by cybersecurity, infrastructure, and cloud teams during solution design. They identified key challenges such as aging systems, system disparity, data inaccuracy, lack of ownership, regulatory constraints, and poor alignment across business units, which often result in silos and redundant tools. The absence of standardized terminology and a heavy focus on technology without organizational alignment were also critical barriers.

Financial decision-makers were seen as cautious, approving investments only when tied to clear business cases and measurable value. SMEs stressed that cloud technology is the preferred platform for big data due to its scalability and agility. However, many business leaders struggle to use real-time analytics without proper training and default to outdated reporting methods.

Furthermore, SMEs agreed that data should be managed as a product, not a project, and is a foundational pillar of digital transformation, feeding into AI and ML. The organizational culture will shift as big data adoption influences decision-making, processes, and workforce needs. Lastly, there is a strong call for greater innovation, predictive analytics, and structured support for physician engagement, acknowledging varying levels of data proficiency. Interview insights were consistent with findings from prior case studies.

REFERENCES

Dworkin, S. L. (2012). Sample size policy for qualitative studies using in-depth interviews. *Archives of Sexual Behavior, 41*(6), 1319–1320. https://doi.org/10.1007/s10508-012-0016-6

Gartner. (2019). *Fusion teams: A new model for digital delivery*. https://www.gartner.com/cn/documents/3955908/fusion-teams-a-new-model-for-digital-delivery

Leung, L. (2015). Validity, reliability, and generalizability in qualitative research. *Journal of Family Medicine and Primary Care, 4*(3), 324–327. https://doi.org/10.4103/2249-4863.161306

Lincoln, Y. S., & Guba, E. G. (1985). *Naturalistic Inquiry*. Sage Publications.

Maier, M. W. (1996). Developments in system architecting. In *Proceedings of ICECCS'96: 2nd IEEE International Conference on Engineering of Complex Computer Systems* (pp. 56–61). IEEE.

Pace, D. K., & Sheehan, J. (2002). Subject matter expert (SME)/peer use in M&S V&V. In *Foundations for the V&V in the 21st Century Workshop (Foundations 2002)*. Johns Hopkins University Applied Physics Laboratory.

Phillips, J. J., Buzachero, V., Phillips, P., & Phillips, Z. (2013). *Measuring ROI in Healthcare: Tools and Techniques to Measure the Impact and ROI in Healthcare Improvement Projects and Programs*. McGraw-Hill Professional.

Steiner, R. (1998). 4.1.3 System architectures and evolvability: Definitions and perspective. In *Proceedings of the 8th Annual International Symposium of the International Council on Systems Engineering (INCOSE)*. (Vol. 8, No. 1, pp. 137–141). Vancouver, British Columbia, Canada, from July 26–30, 1998.

Teter, M. D. (2014). Applying subject matter expertise (SME) elicitation techniques to TRAC studies. No. TRACMTR14036. In *TRAC-TR-14-025*. U.S. Army Training and Doctrine Command Analysis Center.

Whittemore, R., Chase, S. K., & Mandle, C. L. (2001). Validity in qualitative research. *Qualitative Health Research*, *11*(4), 522–537. https://doi.org/10.1177/104973201129119299

Yin, R. K. (2009). *Case Study Research: Design and Methods* (4th ed., Vol. 5). Sage Publications.

Yusoff, M. S. B. (2019). ABC of content validation and content validity index calculation. *Education in Medicine Journal*, *11*(2), 49–54. https://doi.org/10.21315/eimj2019.11.2.6

Conclusion and Future Vision

6

As healthcare enters an era of digital transformation, data proliferation, and intelligent automation, organizations must reevaluate how they harness and manage information to drive outcomes. This book introduced a comprehensive, system-level framework for leveraging big data in healthcare, underpinned by six interconnected pillars: Organization, People, Processes, Data, Technology, and Outcomes. These pillars were not chosen arbitrarily; they emerged from research methodology, literature review, gap analysis, and real-world case validation. Each pillar supports a healthcare system's strategic, operational, and clinical functions, striving to adapt and thrive in a data-intensive environment.

This concluding chapter builds upon the previous discussions by synthesizing key lessons and projecting them into the future of digital health. It evaluates how each framework element must evolve to support long-term transformation and sustainability. The emphasis is on practical alignment with emerging trends in health IT, governance, artificial intelligence, and patient-centered care.

6.1 LESSONS LEARNED FROM THIS JOURNEY

This journey has shown that transforming healthcare with big data is not just about technology but coordination, clarity of purpose, and strategic alignment. Success depends on having a shared vision, strong leadership, and a commitment to using data in ways that directly support patient care, operational efficiency, and informed decision-making.

DOI: 10.1201/9781003610731-6

We also learned that integration matters. Analytics must be embedded into daily routines and adapted to real-world healthcare environments. Systems need to be flexible and responsive to ongoing changes, including regulations, data formats, and clinical workflows. Projects connected to these practical realities are more likely to generate real impact and long-term adoption.

Finally, this journey reminded us that transformation is continuous. Building trust in data, refining processes based on feedback, and addressing ethical and privacy concerns are all essential. The most effective systems evolve from experience and adapt to new challenges, keeping patient outcomes and organizational resilience at the center of their progress.

6.1.1 Organization: Enabling Adaptive Governance

Healthcare organizations must embrace a paradigm shift in governance that recognizes data as a strategic asset and a core capability. The move from traditional hierarchies to adaptive, data-driven structures will be critical for future-readiness. Chief Data Officers (CDOs) and analytics steering committees must be empowered to lead data strategies, set standards, and align initiatives with institutional goals. Strategic imperatives such as value-based care, patient-centered delivery, and digital front-door initiatives must be supported by clearly defined data governance policies, accountability frameworks, and integrated oversight.

Additionally, organizations must create feedback loops that leverage analytics to assess performance and adapt policies in real-time. The governance model must encourage interdepartmental coordination, enabling cross-functional data collaboration among finance, operations, clinical, and regulatory stakeholders. Partnerships with academic, regulatory, and private sector entities must also be part of an ecosystem approach to continuous improvement and innovation.

6.1.2 People: Empowering the Data-Centric Workforce

Human capital is the catalyst for transformation. As healthcare embraces a digital future, its workforce must be reskilled and designed to meet the demands of big data and analytics. Clinical, operational, and administrative staff must be empowered with data literacy training, tools for self-service analytics, and cultural shifts that value evidence-based decision-making.

Data teams—composed of data scientists, engineers, analysts, and business translators—must be structured and strategically positioned to support enterprise-wide needs. The CDO should lead efforts to define job roles, recruit talent, and foster a community of practice that promotes innovation, ethics, and collaboration. Employee engagement programs should integrate analytics into daily tasks, making data a natural extension of everyone's workflow.

Moreover, incentives should be tied to data-driven performance metrics, and departments should be encouraged to share use cases, lessons learned, and impact stories to cultivate a learning organization. The future healthcare workforce must adopt digital tools and become co-creators of value using these tools.

6.1.3 Processes: Operationalizing Intelligence Across the Continuum

Data must be embedded into every aspect of clinical and operational processes to unlock its full value. Process redesign enables workflow alignment with strategic goals by using tools like SIPOC-R and process mapping. Automation powered by big data—such as auto-population of clinical documentation, algorithmic KPI extraction, or AI-assisted diagnoses—can reduce administrative burden and enhance clinical accuracy.

Healthcare organizations must also build dynamic processes that adapt to incoming data. For example, care management protocols can be adjusted in real time based on patient risk scores, and staffing decisions can be dynamically rebalanced using predictive analytics. Processes should be streamlined to facilitate data ingestion, cleansing, analysis, and feedback loops. Additionally, digital process ownership should be assigned, with accountability for quality and efficiency at every touchpoint.

Standard operating procedures must be redefined in the context of digital health, ensuring that data flows securely and efficiently across systems while maintaining interoperability. Inter-organizational processes, such as data sharing with external providers, payers, and regulatory bodies, must also be optimized and continuously evaluated.

6.1.4 Data: Ensuring Completeness, Governance, and Utility

Data is the core asset of the digital health enterprise. Data must be timely, complete, high-quality, and ethically managed to enable transformation. The framework promotes a comprehensive approach to data management that includes governance structures, lifecycle policies, and stewardship roles.

Data sources must be expanded beyond traditional EMR/EHR systems to include patient-generated data, social determinants of health, wearable device streams, imaging data, and structured/unstructured clinical notes. These diverse formats must be integrated through robust data pipelines supporting real-time analytics. Participating in national initiatives such as Health Information Exchanges (HIEs) and leveraging platforms like i2b2 or n2c2 can enhance data comprehensiveness and analytical reach.

Implementing data quality assurance programs and metadata management systems is equally critical. These initiatives build trust in the data, essential for making impactful decisions. Privacy, security, and compliance must be rigorously maintained, particularly in the context of HIPAA, GDPR, and other relevant frameworks.

6.1.5 Technology: Building a Scalable, Agile Ecosystem

Digital transformation is inseparable from the underlying technology stack. Future-ready healthcare enterprises must invest in scalable, cloud-based infrastructures that support high-volume, high-velocity, and high-variety data. Architectural design must emphasize modularity, elasticity, and real-time capabilities.

Integration tools should support API-driven interoperability and accommodate structured, semi-structured, and unstructured data. Big data platforms must have security, auditing, data masking, and encryption capabilities. AI/ML engines, voice recognition systems, and natural language processing tools are essential to transform unstructured inputs into actionable insights.

Visualization layers like dynamic dashboards and interactive scorecards should be user-friendly and accessible across mobile and desktop environments. Additionally, technology procurement should be guided by frameworks such as MoSCoW prioritization, ensuring alignment with operational goals and regulatory needs.

Strategic partnerships with technology vendors must be cultivated to ensure ongoing innovation and alignment with emerging standards and compliance requirements. Composable digital architecture enables organizations to remain agile and respond to new challenges without major infrastructure overhauls.

6.1.6 Outcomes: Achieving Strategic, Clinical, and Financial Impact

Ultimately, the framework must demonstrate measurable improvements in outcomes. At the clinical level, big data analytics should reduce medical errors, prevent readmissions, enhance diagnostic accuracy, and personalize care delivery. Business outcomes include improved revenue cycle performance, optimized resource allocation, and strengthened regulatory compliance.

Performance measurements must be embedded in every layer of the organization, from Balanced Scorecards and KPIs to star ratings and quality certifications. Dashboards should present real-time updates that facilitate proactive interventions rather than retrospective corrections. Organizations must benchmark their outcomes against peers, using platforms like CMS quality ratings, Leapfrog, and HIMSS Digital Maturity models.

Furthermore, the patient experience must be improved through seamless digital interactions, personalized communication, and timely access to care. As value-based care models mature, healthcare organizations must demonstrate that their investments in big data lead to better outcomes at lower costs.

The framework proposed in this book is more than a theoretical construct—it is a strategic roadmap for the future of digital health. By integrating systems thinking, industrial engineering principles, and advanced data technologies, healthcare organizations can transform into intelligent, agile enterprises capable of thriving in a rapidly evolving ecosystem. The journey toward digital maturity is complex, but the rewarding qualities, efficiency, equity, and sustainability are profound.

6.2 THE FUTURE TRAJECTORY

This section explores the future trajectory in the era of Healthcare 4.0, examining how trends such as generative AI, ethical data governance, and intelligent automation will shape the next generation of solutions. We contextualize the framework within ongoing transformations and offer forward-looking strategies for healthcare leaders navigating this unprecedented acceleration (Singhal et al., 2025).

6.2.1 The Generative AI Revolution in Healthcare

Generative AI marks a significant leap forward from traditional AI models. While previous systems primarily focused on classification and prediction, generative models such as large language models (LLMs) can synthesize novel content, translate complex data, and interact conversationally with users. In healthcare, these capabilities are redefining the boundaries of what is possible.

Health systems and payers are deploying LLMs to automate prior authorizations, generate clinical documentation, personalize patient communication, and even support diagnostics. These models can produce discharge summaries from clinical notes, predict care pathways, and simulate complex clinical scenarios, offering timesaving and quality-enhancing benefits (Singhal et al., 2024).

However, integrating generative AI also introduces new complexities. Hallucination risks, liability concerns, and interpretability issues necessitate rigorous governance. Embedding these tools into the existing framework demands extensions to the "Technology" and "People" pillars, including clinician retraining, transparency measures, and human-in-the-loop validation systems.

6.2.2 Ethical Imperatives: Trust, Transparency, and Accountability

Ethical considerations become paramount as the healthcare industry embraces more powerful AI systems. Deploying big data and AI technologies in clinical and operational workflows has profound implications for equity, fairness, and patient safety.

Ethical AI frameworks must account for:

- **Bias mitigation:** Training data often reflects historical disparities. AI tools must undergo continuous auditing to prevent perpetuating bias.

- **Explainability:** Clinicians must understand why an algorithm made a decision. Tools such as SHAP, LIME, and counterfactual explanations can aid interpretability.
- **Privacy and consent:** With new data sources such as social media and wearable devices, consent models must evolve. Federated learning is emerging as a privacy-preserving method to train models without centralizing data.
- **Accountability:** There must be clear responsibility chains when AI decisions lead to adverse outcomes.

These ethical elements must be baked into the design of AI systems, not bolted on afterward. The framework underscored the necessity of governance boards, interdisciplinary oversight, and auditability. Future-ready frameworks will treat ethics as a continuous process rather than a fixed checklist.

6.2.3 Digital Payers and the Acceleration of Value-Based Models

The transformation of healthcare payers signals important changes for the entire healthcare system. Payers rapidly embrace digital technologies, using AI to streamline claims management, automate member services, and improve cost forecasting. Generative AI further enhances these capabilities by enabling the summarization of clinical records and providing natural language responses to policyholder inquiries (Carrus et al., 2023). Value-based care models will increasingly depend on AI-driven insights. Predictive analytics can identify high-risk members, personalize preventive interventions, and reduce avoidable admissions. To support this, payers and providers must co-create interoperable data ecosystems.

For our framework, this trend reinforces the need for:

- interoperability across institutions,
- embedded analytics in operational workflows, and
- governance models that span payer-provider boundaries.

6.2.4 From Smart Hospitals to Ambient Healthcare

The acceleration of Healthcare 4.0 is transforming care environments. Hospitals are becoming smart ecosystems powered by Internet of Things

(IoT) devices, edge computing, and real-time analytics. Patient rooms now feature voice-activated systems, biometric monitoring, and AI-driven alert mechanisms.

This shift is marked by innovations such as digital twins, continuous virtual care, and predictive staffing tools (Vallée, 2024). These technologies support more personalized, preventive, and proactive care models that enhance outcomes across the healthcare system. This evolution demands enhancements to the framework, such as:

- integration of edge analytics for latency-sensitive applications,
- adaptive process modeling to accommodate continuous data streams, and
- clinical workflow redesign with digital co-pilots.

6.2.5 Strategic Recommendations for Stakeholders

Based on insights from the literature and recent developments, the following recommendations are proposed for healthcare stakeholders aiming to operationalize the framework in the era of Healthcare 4.0:

1. **Build modular, federated architectures** to balance privacy with interoperability.
2. **Pilot generative AI use cases** in controlled settings with clinician supervision.
3. **Form interdisciplinary AI ethics committees** with representation from patients, clinicians, data scientists, and legal experts.
4. **Adopt explainability standards** for all predictive or generative models in clinical care.
5. **Redesign clinical workflows** around digital augmentation tools rather than treating AI as an add-on.
6. **Develop competency models** for upskilling the workforce in data literacy and AI utilization.
7. **Measure and benchmark AI outcomes** using KPIs reflecting process efficiency and care equity.

These strategies ensure technological adoption, organizational readiness, and cultural alignment (Pesqueira et al., 2025).

6.3 TOWARD A RESILIENT, INTELLIGENT HEALTHCARE SYSTEM

As we transition into an era increasingly defined by digital augmentation, the convergence of big data, Artificial Intelligence (AI), and healthcare demands a deliberate integration of technology, ethics, and human expertise. The framework presented throughout this book offers a foundational blueprint for orchestrating this integration, positioning healthcare organizations to adapt intelligently and act in the face of accelerating complexity.

However, this journey is not static. Future iterations of the framework must continuously evolve, absorbing insights from real-world deployments, embracing emergent technologies, and responding to shifting societal needs and regulatory landscapes. A healthcare system's true resilience lies in its ability to learn, adapt, and transform with agility.

To fulfill Healthcare 4.0's vision, organizations must move beyond isolated innovations and adopt holistic, patient-centered strategies. This includes embedding ethical AI into clinical and operational workflows, fostering cross-sector data interoperability, and equipping healthcare professionals with intelligent, context-aware tools that enhance—not replace—their judgment.

By aligning technological advancement with ethical governance, inclusive design, and collaborative leadership, we can build healthcare systems that are more efficient and precise, equitable, transparent, and responsive. The path forward is not simply about adopting new tools but about cultivating new capabilities, partnerships, and mindsets to support a resilient, intelligent, and truly human-centered future.

REFERENCES

Carrus, B., Chowdhary, S., Fleron, A., & Groch, N. (2023). *Rewiring Healthcare Payers: A Guide to Digital and AI Transformation.* McKinsey & Company.

Pesqueira, A., Sousa, M. J., Pereira, R., & Schwendinger, M. (2025). Designing and implementing SMILE: An AI-driven platform for enhancing clinical decision-making in mental health and neurodivergence management. *Computational and Structural Biotechnology Journal*, *27*, 785–803. https://doi.org/10.1016/j.csbj.2025.02.022

Singhal, S., Patel, N., & Jain, A. (2025). *What to Expect in US Healthcare in 2025 and Beyond*. McKinsey & Company.

Singhal, S., Patel, N., Jain, A., & Shah, A. (2024). *Generative AI in Healthcare: Current Trends and Future Outlook*: Vol. Version 3. McKinsey & Company.

Vallée, A. (2024). Challenges and directions for digital twin implementation in oto-rhinolaryngology. *European Archives of Oto-Rhino-Laryngology*, *281*(11), 6155–6159. https://doi.org/10.1007/s00405-024-08662-5

Index

Note: Bold page numbers refer to tables and Italic page numbers refer to figures.

I

K

M

N

O

P

Q

R

S

T

V